the **Family**

g.i. diet

**THE HEALTHY, GREEN-LIGHT WAY
TO MANAGE WEIGHT FOR YOUR ENTIRE FAMILY**

RICK GALLOP
& DR. RUTH GALLOP

RANDOM HOUSE CANADA

To our sons, Michael, Stephen and David, for both their joyful tolerance and enthusiastic involvement in Dad's family food experiments over the years

Copyright © 2005 Green Light Foods Inc.

All rights reserved under International and Pan-American Copyright Conventions. No part of this book may be reproduced in any form or by any electronic or mechanical means, including information storage and retrieval systems, without permission in writing from the publisher, except by a reviewer, who may quote brief passages in a review. Published in 2005 by Random House Canada, a division of Random House of Canada Limited. Distributed in Canada by Random House of Canada Limited.

Random House Canada and colophon are trademarks.

www.randomhouse.ca

LIBRARY AND ARCHIVES CANADA CATALOGUING IN PUBLICATION

Gallop, Rick
    The family G.I. diet : the healthy green-light way to manage weight for your entire family / Rick Gallop and Ruth Gallop.

Includes index.
ISBN-13: 978-0-679-31321-2
ISBN-10: 0-679-31321-4

    1. Glycemic index. 2. Reducing diets. 3. Family—Health and hygiene. I. Gallop, Ruth Margaret, 1943– II. Title.

RM222.2.G33 2005   613.2'5   C2005-903761-X

Printed and bound in Canada

10 9 8 7 6 5 4 3 2 1

Contents

Foreword

You've got to start somewhere, but there's no point starting a diet unless you intend to be successful. That's what this book is all about: helping you succeed in reaching your goal of a much healthier lifestyle, not just in the short term but from now on. And it's not just for you but for your entire family.

What's so special about this diet book? Why follow its advice rather than the suggestions found in all the other diet books on the shelf? The G.I. Diet is nutritionally sound and scientifically based. It takes complex nutritional concepts and makes them easy to understand and put into practice with a creative traffic light system. *The G.I. Diet* offers no gimmicks or quick fixes. It is sustainable. It is transforming.

This book, *The Family G.I. Diet*, takes the proven, best-selling concepts of the original *G.I. Diet* one important step further: it addresses the entire family. It allows spouses to support one another in the difficult tasks of weight control and eating properly. It deals with age and gender differences. It encourages parents to serve as role models for their children. It makes parents aware of the various behavioural stages of childhood that must be appreciated to improve that most basic of activities, the family meal.

The author, Rick Gallop, is a very special person. He is bright, articulate and innovative. Rick's credentials for writing a diet book are a bit unusual. He is not a nutritionist, nor is he a physician. But for fifteen years, he served as president of the Heart and Stroke Foundation of Ontario. He developed a passion for promoting healthy lifestyles that reduce the risk of cardiovascular disease and its devastating consequences. Rick became frustrated at the high failure rates associated with most diet plans. So, true to his character, he sought to devise a better diet method. And he did.

Ultimately, improving how you and your loved ones live is up to you. If you need some help with this, *The Family G.I. Diet* is a wonderful guide that will make your entire family feel better and stay healthier. Enjoy the book and enjoy each other.

Norman R. Saunders, MD, FRCP(C)
Department of Pediatrics,
University of Toronto

What is special about being a family doctor is having the chance to accompany a family through many of life's stages. Where else in medicine does one get to witness children progressing from birth to adolescence and on to adulthood, or middle-aged patients moving on to grapple with retirement or deteriorating health? I have been practising for over twenty years, and the infants I once cared for are now expecting their own children, the young mothers whom I once commiserated with about their sleepless nights are now losing sleep because of hot flashes. As time has passed I have also witnessed the impact of information technology, which has transformed passive patients into active health care advocates who are interested in maintaining health and preventing illness.

At any life stage, nutrition is a primary concern. For this reason, I have welcomed the G.I. Diet as an excellent resource when counselling patients. Diets in general have been anathema to me, because by their very nature they have a start point and an end point, with consequent rebounding and accumulation of even more weight. The G.I. approach is more of a lifestyle than a diet, and it is sustainable because it is based on sound scientific principles. Organizing foods in categories based on the colours of a traffic light provides a straightforward system of eating that anyone can grasp and apply.

In *The Family G.I. Diet,* Rick Gallop takes the program further by recommending practices to last a lifetime. There is excellent advice on including children in grocery shopping and meal preparation, plus setting clear but flexible limits regarding mealtimes and snacks. One significant piece of information the Gallops share is that it takes ten to fifteen exposures to a new food for a child to accept it. This means parents should not give up introducing their children to vegetables if they initially refuse them. The book also emphasizes the importance of exercise, especially for seniors. This advice is supported by the World Health Organization's preliminary findings that eating well and exercising not only extend one's lifespan but also prevent infirmity.

The G.I. Diet is a weight-loss program that I am able to endorse as I see its results with my own eyes. Patients thank me for recommending the diet to them because they've lost weight and feel more energetic than ever. Embarking on this program has immediate health benefits and also teaches us life lessons about staying well.

Pauline Pariser, M.Asc, MD, CCFP, CFCP
Assistant Professor,
Department of Family and Community Medicine,
University of Toronto

Introduction

My first book, *The G.I. Diet,* was published in 2002 and quickly became the most successful Canadian diet book ever, with more than one and a half million copies sold worldwide. It is currently available in fifteen countries, in a dozen different languages, and it made *The New York Times* bestseller list. The Canadian Diabetes Association rated the G.I. Diet as the first choice among today's leading diets— and there are a lot of them to choose from now! But my greatest delight has been the enormous number of reader e-mails I've received. I had no idea that the book would generate such a flood of responses, and I was amazed to hear about all the ways in which this new approach to eating has actually changed people's lives. I've heard from tens of thousands of readers, in messages that are personal, thoughtful, supportive—and frequently ecstatic!

It was this feedback that encouraged me to embark on this new book, *The Family G.I. Diet.* Why focus on the family? The first reason is that most of the correspondence I've received has been from women. And despite all the changes in family life, for better or worse most women still play the role of chief shopper, cook and gatekeeper for their family's health and nutrition. At the same time, women, as well as men, are working longer hours outside the house. They just can't devote a lot of their time to "managing" the way the family eats, too. One of their biggest challenges is figuring out how to prepare a different set of diet meals for themselves while cooking for the rest of the family. How can they control their own weight, meet the needs and culinary whims of the rest of the family and somehow avoid becoming a short-order cook?

There's another consideration as well. Men and women have different nutritional needs, depending on their stage of life and hormonal factors. A woman expecting twins won't have the same appetite and nutritional demands as the elderly grandfather who might be sharing the dinner table with her. Menopause also brings its own metabolic changes and nutritional shifts for women. And teenagers may have a strange concept of what constitutes a "hearty breakfast." My wife, Ruth, and I have raised three children—one of them a vegetarian—so we're well aware of the challenges of feeding a family whose members' appetites and tastes vary.

Women are not only concerned about their own weight, but they also worry about their overweight spouses, partners and children. Is your partner overweight? Since just under 56 percent of Canadian men are either in that category or officially obese, there is a good chance that this is the case. (See the Body Mass Index on pages 34–35 to see if he qualifies.)

And you've probably been reading about the alarming increase in childhood obesity. According to recent studies, 37 percent of Canadian children between two and eleven years old are overweight. At the same time, you don't want your children—especially your daughters—to become obsessed with weight loss and body image. What you *do* want is to establish healthy patterns of eating that keep your children fit and energetic, not only as they are growing up but for the rest of their lives. What you *don't* want to do is cater to their every whim by cooking three different meals every night. You can't really blame kids for their cravings. With so many processed, over-advertised, high-fat snack foods available, they are simply following the path of least resistance. We need to give them appealing options.

So I could see that a family approach to the G.I. Diet would be helpful, and the result is this book, *The Family G.I. Diet.* I persuaded my wife, Ruth, who is professor emeritus of the faculties of nursing and medicine at the University of Toronto, to provide a female perspective, as well as to share her experience in women's health issues and behavioural research. She wrote chapter six, which outlines the special nutritional needs of women from menarche to menopause and beyond, and gave valuable information on feeding children at various stages of their life. Together we talk about how to follow the G.I. Diet along with spouses, partners, toddlers and teenagers. We give you help with shopping, meal planning and lunch packing, and have included fifty new delicious recipes that are G.I. versions of family favourites. We address the special needs of seniors, who are often neglected in other diet books, and help you use nutrition to reduce your family's risk of heart disease, stroke, diabetes, most cancers and even degenerative conditions like Alzheimer's. The evidence from medical research is overwhelming that weight management and diet are the most effective ways to reduce your risk of these life-threatening diseases. So the G.I. Diet is not just about losing weight simply and painlessly; it's also about a permanent gain in quality of life.

On the G.I. Diet, you won't go hungry or feel deprived, and you will never have to count another calorie or carb. I'm a firm believer that a diet shouldn't have to involve higher math! How is this possible? The keys are simplicity and nutritional balance. With its emphasis on fruits, vegetables, whole grains, low-fat dairy products, lean meat and seafood, the G.I. Diet is an ideal way for the whole family to eat, whether weight control is an issue or not. And if you or your partner needs to shed five pounds or fifty, *The Family G.I. Diet* will show both of you how to eat more healthily and lose weight from the same menu.

For more information on the G.I. Diet, a free subscription to my quarterly newsletter and details about how to contact me with your comments and suggestions, please visit my website at **www.gidiet.com**. I would love to hear from you.

PART I

The G.I. Diet Program

CHAPTER ONE

Why Do You Want to Lose Weight?

Do you want to lose ten pounds or a hundred? Perhaps you just want to drop a dress size or two while you help your overweight partner lose a significant amount of weight. It's important to look at the reasons why you or members of your family want to lose weight; your answer will have a lot to do with your motivation to start and, more important, to stay the course with your new way of eating.

Let's look at the most common reasons why people want to lose weight and see how they reflect your own.

1. I want to look better.

Judging from the correspondence I have received— 20,000 emails and counting—the day when people discover that they have to dig out their "skinny" pants again is at least as rewarding as seeing the numbers fall on the scale. Most of us would rather shop for clothes that flatter and show off the body rather than resort to camouflage. It's a powerful motivator to walk into a room and hear a friend ask, "Have you lost weight? You look terrific." I've sold more books based on word of mouth—people asking *G.I. Diet* readers how they lost their weight—than through any other marketing strategy.

But losing weight is not just about trying to live up to unreachable, red-carpet standards of beauty or thinness; it's about feeling at ease in your body and liking what you see in the mirror. Weight loss boosts self-esteem and confidence, which in turn makes it easier to maintain new

Dear Rick,
I lost 85 pounds in 22 weeks, but the real news is what a difference that weight change has made to my appearance. I went to a family wedding last weekend and was embarrassed by the attention I got. The room seemed to stop and gasp when I walked into the reception! I lost count of how many people asked what happened, told me how good I looked, asked what diet I was on and how much weight I had lost. By the way, my cholesterol and other health stats are fantastic! There is certainly no more rewarding personal journey than transforming your body into what you always wanted it to be. I can't begin to express how valuable the G.I. Diet has been to making this happen.
Derek

eating habits. It's amazing the difference the loss of just a few pounds can make, not only to how you look in your clothes but to how you feel about yourself.

2. I want to feel more energetic and less lethargic.

Perhaps what I hear about most frequently from readers, other than the thrill of losing pounds or going down a dress size, is the surge of energy that comes with a lighter, healthier body. I witnessed a dramatic demonstration of the kind of burden extra weight can be just the other day. My wife and I had just completed some house renovations to suit our empty-nest lifestyle, and as we were restoring some order, I asked Ruth to carry a couple of 20-pound dumbbells up a flight of stairs to my new workout room. She could only get them to the first floor landing before she had to put them down again. "How do people who are 40 pounds overweight get around, let alone climb stairs?" she wondered. And 40 pounds of extra weight is not something you can just put down when you want to. Imagine the energy that goes into carrying those pounds! That's the energy that will be available to you again if you shed the excess weight.

Readers also tell me about the delight they experience when they find themselves able to do more exercise and to enjoy activities they haven't participated in since their teens. If regaining your former energy and vitality is important to you, you'll receive constant motivation as your new, lighter body rejoices in its recently acquired freedom to run, swim, play squash, or engage in any activity you may have given up for "lack of energy."

3. I want to be healthier, and I want to help my family become healthier.

Although health may not be your primary reason for losing weight, it is ultimately the most important one. Excess weight and poor diet are by far the most critical factors in increasing your chances of developing major diseases that can either undermine your quality of life or drastically shorten it. These include heart disease, stroke, cancer, diabetes and Alzheimer's. Of course, genes play a role in your risk of these diseases too, but anyone who is overweight and undernourished is putting herself at increased risk for these conditions. The prospect of a long life, especially one free of pain, disability and disease, is a powerful motivator.

Keeping in mind these three incentives—looking and feeling better, enjoying greater energy and improving your overall health—will go a long way in helping you stick to the G.I. Diet and will open up a whole new chapter in your life. But if losing weight has so many obvious benefits, why is the prevalence of overweight and obesity steadily increasing, especially as hundreds of new diet books flood the stores each year? Well, the fact is that most diets don't work. And the reason they fail is that people don't stay on them. Why do they give up? I'm sure the following explanations will be familiar to you.

Why Diets Don't Work

1. Most diets leave you feeling hungry, weak and deprived. You stagger through the day with a grumbling stomach, but sooner or later you cave and order a pizza with double cheese. Feeling perpetually hungry is the primary reason that people give up on their diet.

2. The diet is too complicated and time-consuming to follow. You spend each day weighing and measuring food, calculating carbs or calories and keeping food diaries. Perhaps this is fun initially, but then it all just becomes a burden. You're too busy to follow a diet that feels more like a math exam.

3. You feel bad. Many diets cut out essential nutrients, leaving you feeling lethargic and concerned about your health. Is it little wonder people give up?

Why Have We Gotten So Fat?

Nearly 56 percent of Canadians are overweight, and our obesity rate has doubled over the past twenty years. The rate of increase in obesity in children is even worse. So what's happening to us? Why, in a relatively short time, have we gained so much weight?

It's not as if we lack awareness of weight issues. There are shelves of books and racks of magazines with cover stories on diets and fitness regimens. The media have latched onto the "obesity epidemic" with a fervour—fat is big news these days.

But the reason for our collective weight crisis is actually quite simple: we're consuming more calories than we're expending, and the resulting surplus is stored around our waists, hips and thighs as fat. (Maybe it's found a nice spot on your upper arms, too.) There's no mystery here. But to understand *why* we seem to be consuming more calories, we need to get back to basics and look at the three fundamental elements of our diet: carbohydrates, fats and proteins. I'm sure you've heard about these characters. We need to understand how they work together, whether we're in the process of getting fat or thin, and the role they play in our digestive system.

We'll start with carbohydrates, since the popularity of low-carbohydrate diets like the Atkins program has made them a hot topic and given them a bad rap. They've been so much in the news over the past few years that a new word has entered the language: "carbs." Though they've been blamed for all our weight problems, their role in weight control has really been misunderstood.

Carbohydrates

Carbohydrates are a necessary part of a healthy diet. They are rich in fibre, vitamins and minerals, including antioxidants, which we now know play an important role in the prevention of heart disease and cancer. Carbohydrates are also the primary source of energy for our bodies. They are found in grains, vegetables, fruits, legumes (beans) and dairy products.

Here is how carbs work: when you eat an orange or a bagel, your body digests the carbohydrates in the food and turns them into glucose, which provides you with energy. The glucose dissolves in your bloodstream and then travels to the parts of your body that use energy, such as your muscles and brain. So carbs are critical to everyone's health. What is important to realize when managing weight, however, is that not all carbs are made the same.

Some carbohydrates break down into glucose in our digestive system at a slow and steady rate, gradually releasing their nutrients and keeping us feeling full and satisfied. Others break down rapidly, spiking our glucose levels and then disappearing quickly, leaving us feeling hungry again. For example, old-fashioned, large-flake oatmeal and cornflakes are both carbohydrates, but we all know the difference between eating a bowl of the oatmeal for breakfast and eating a bowl of cornflakes. The oatmeal stays with you—it "sticks to your ribs" as my mother used to say—whereas your stomach starts rumbling an hour after eating the cornflakes, propelling you toward your next snack or meal. If throughout the course of a day, then, you are eating carbs that break down rapidly, like cornflakes, as opposed to those that break down slowly, you are going to be eating more and, as a result, will begin to put on weight. If, however, you start eating carbs that break down slowly, like old-fashioned oatmeal, you will eat less and begin to lose weight. Selecting the right type of carb is key to achieving your optimum energy and weight. But how do you know which carbohydrate is the right type and which isn't?

Well the first clue is the amount of processing that the food has undergone. The more a food is processed beyond its natural, fibrous state, the less processing your body has to do to digest it. And the quicker you digest the food, the sooner you feel hungry again. This helps explain why the number of Canadian adults who are overweight has grown exponentially over the last fifty years. A hundred years ago, most of the food people ate came straight from the farm to the dinner table. Lack of refrigeration and scant knowledge of food chemistry meant that most food remained in its original state. However, advances in science, along with the migration of many women out of the kitchen and into the workforce, lead to a revolution in prepared foods. Everything became geared to speed and simplicity of preparation. The giant food companies—Kraft, Kellogg's, Del Monte, Nestlé, etc.—were born. We happily began spending more money for the convenience of prepared, processed, packaged, canned, frozen and bottled food. The Kraft Dinner era had begun.

It was during this period that the miller's traditional wind and water mills were replaced with high-speed steel rolling mills, which stripped away most of the key nutrients, including the bran, fibre and wheat germ (which could spoil), to produce a talcum-like powder: today's white flour. This fine white flour is the basic ingredient for most of our breads and cereals, as well as for baked goods and snacks such as cookies, muffins, crackers and pretzels. Walk through any supermarket and you will be surrounded by towering stacks of these flour-based processed products. And we're eating more and more of these foods; over the past three decades, our consumption of grain has increased by 50 percent. Our bodies are paying the price for this radical change in eating habits.

The second clue in determining whether a carbohydrate is the right type is the amount of fibre it contains. Fibre, in simple terms, provides low-calorie filler. It does double duty, in fact: it literally fills up your stomach, so you feel satiated; and your body takes much longer to break it down, so it stays with you longer and slows down the digestive process. There are two forms of fibre: soluble and insoluble. Soluble fibre is found in carbs like oatmeal, beans, barley and citrus fruits, and has been shown to lower blood cholesterol levels. Insoluble fibre is important for normal bowel function and is typically found in whole wheat breads and cereals and most vegetables.

There are two other important components that inhibit the rapid breakdown of food in our digestive system, and they are fats and protein. Let's look at fats first.

Fats

Fat, like fibre, acts as a brake in the digestive process. When combined with other foods, fat becomes a barrier to digestive juices. It also signals the brain that you are satisfied and do not require more food. Does this mean that we should eat all the fat we want? Definitely not!

Though fat is essential for a nutritious diet, containing various key elements that are crucial to the digestive process, cell development and overall health, it also contains twice the number of calories per gram as carbohydrates and protein. If you decide to "just add peanut butter" to your otherwise disciplined regime, it doesn't take much of it—two tablespoons—to spike your total calorie count. As well, once you eat fat, your body is a genius at hanging onto it and refusing to let it go. This is because fat is how the body stores reserve supplies of energy, usually around the waist, hips and thighs. Fat is money in the bank as far as the body is concerned—a rainy-day investment for when you have to call up extra energy. This clever system originally helped our ancestors survive during periods of famine. The problem today is that we don't live with cycles of feast and famine—it's more like feast, and then feast again! But the body's eagerness for fat continues, along with its reluctance to give it up.

This is why losing weight is so difficult: your body does everything it can to persuade you to eat more fat. How? Through fat's capacity to make things taste good. So it's not just you who thinks that juicy steaks, chocolate cake and rich ice cream taste better than a bean sprout. That's the fat content of cake and steak talking.

Sorry to say, there's no getting around it: if you want to lose weight, you have to watch your fat consumption. In addition, you need to be concerned about the type of fat you eat. Many fats are harmful to your health. There are four types of fat: the best, the good, the bad and the really ugly. The "really ugly" fats are potentially the most dangerous, and they lurk in many of our most popular snack foods. They are vegetable oils that have been heat-treated to make them thicken—the trans fats you've been hearing so much about in the media lately. They raise the amount of LDL, or bad, cholesterol, in our bodies while lowering the amount of HDL, or good, cholesterol, which protects us from heart disease. As a result they boost our cholesterol level, which thickens our arteries and causes heart attack and stroke. So avoid using trans fats, like vegetable shortening and hard margarine, and avoid packaged snack foods, baked goods, crackers and cereals that contain them. (You can spot them by checking labels for "hydrogenated" or "partially hydrogenated" oils.)

The "bad" fats are called saturated fats, and almost always come from animal sources. Butter, cheese and meat are all high in saturated fats. There are a couple of others you should be aware of too: coconut oil and palm oil are two vegetable oils that are saturated, and because they are cheap, they are used in many snack foods, especially cookies. Saturated fats are the ones that are solid at room temperature, such as butter or cheese. They elevate your risk of heart disease and Alzheimer's. The evidence is also growing that many cancers, including colon, prostate and breast, are associated with diets high in saturated fats.

The "good" fats are the polyunsaturated ones, and they are cholesterol-free. Most vegetable oils, such as corn and sunflower, fall into this category. What you really *should* be eating, however, are the monounsaturated fats, which actually promote good health. These are the fats found in olives, almonds, and canola and olive oils. Monounsaturated fats have a beneficial effect on cholesterol and are good for your heart. This is one reason why the incidence of heart disease is low in Mediterranean countries, where olive oil is a staple. Although fancy olive oil is expensive, you can enjoy the same health benefits from less costly supermarket brands. It doesn't have to be extra-virgin, double cold pressed.

Another highly beneficial oil that falls into its own category is omega-3, a fatty acid that is found in deep-sea fish, such as salmon, mackerel, albacore tuna and herring, as well as in lake trout, walnuts, and flaxseed and canola oils. Some brands of eggs and liquid eggs also contain omega-3, which can help lower cholesterol and protect your cardiovascular health.

So "good" fats are an important part of a healthy diet and also help slow down digestion. Still, they're fat and they pack a lot of calories. We have to be careful, then, to limit our intake of polyunsaturated fats like almonds and olives when trying to lose weight. Since protein also acts as a brake in the digestive process, let's look at it in more detail.

Protein

Protein is an absolutely essential part of your diet. In fact, you are already half protein: 50 percent of your dry body weight is made up of muscles, organs, skin and hair, all forms of protein. We need this element to build and repair body tissues, and it figures in nearly all metabolic reactions. Protein is also a critical brain food, providing amino acids for the neurotransmitters that relay messages to the brain. This is why it's not a good idea to skip breakfast on the morning of a big meeting or exam. The "brain fog" people experience on some diets is likely the result of diminished protein. Protein is literally food for thought.

The main sources of dietary protein come from animals: meat, seafood, dairy and eggs. Vegetable sources include beans and soy-based products like tofu. Unfortunately, protein sources such as red meat and full-fat dairy products are also high in "bad," or saturated fats, which are harmful to your health. It is important that we get our protein from sources that are low in saturated fats, such as lean meats, skinless poultry, seafood, low-fat dairy products, cholesterol-reduced liquid eggs, and tofu and other soy products. One exceptional source of protein is the humble bean. Beans are a perfect food, really; they're high in protein and fibre, and low in saturated fat. No wonder so many of the world's cuisines have found myriad wonderful ways to cook beans. North Americans need to become more bean savvy. Nuts are another excellent source of protein that are relatively low in fat—as long as you don't eat a whole bowlful.

Protein is much more effective than carbohydrates or fat in satisfying hunger. It will make you feel fuller longer, which is why you should always try to incorporate some protein in every meal and snack. This will help keep you on the ball and feeling satisfied.

Now that we know how carbohydrates, fats and proteins work in our digestive system and what makes us gain weight, let's use the science to put together an eating plan that will take off the extra pounds.

TO SUM UP
- Eat carbohydrates that have not been highly processed and that do not contain highly processed ingredients.
- Eat less fat overall and look for low-fat alternatives to your current diet.
- Eat monounsaturated and polyunsaturated fats only.
- Include some protein in all your meals and snacks.
- Eat only low-fat protein, preferably from both animal and vegetable sources.

CHAPTER TWO

The G.I. Diet

The "G.I." in G.I. Diet stands for glycemic index, which is the basis of this diet (and the only scientific phrase you'll need to know). The glycemic index is the secret to reducing calories and losing weight without going hungry. It measures the speed at which carbohydrates break down in our digestive system and turn into glucose, the body's main source of energy or fuel.

The glycemic index was developed by Dr. David Jenkins, a professor of nutritional sciences at the University of Toronto, when he was researching the impact of different carbohydrates on the blood sugar, or glucose, level of diabetics. He found that certain carbohydrates broke down quickly and flooded the bloodstream with sugar, but others broke down more slowly, only marginally increasing blood sugar levels. The faster a food breaks down, the higher the rating on the glycemic index, which sets sugar at 100 and scores all other foods against that number. These findings were important to diabetics, who could then use the index to identify low-G.I., slow-release foods that would help control their blood sugar levels. Here are some examples of the G.I. ratings of a range of popular foods:

Examples of G.I. Ratings			
High G.I.		**Low G.I.**	
Baguette	95	Orange	44
Cornflakes	84	All-Bran	43
Rice cake	82	Oatmeal	42
Doughnut	76	Spaghetti	41
Bagel	72	Apple	38
Cereal bar	72	Beans	31
Biscuit	69	Plain yogurt	25

What do these G.I. ratings have to do with the numbers on your bathroom scales? Well, it turns out that low-G.I., slow-release foods have a significant impact on our ability to lose weight. As I have explained, when we eat the wrong type of carb, a high-G.I. food, the body quickly digests it and releases a flood of sugar (glucose) into the bloodstream. This gives us a short-term high, but the sugar is just as quickly absorbed by the body, leaving us with a post-sugar slump. We feel lethargic and start looking for our next sugar fix. A fast-food lunch of a double cheeseburger, fries and a Coke delivers a short-term burst of energy, but by mid-afternoon we start feeling tired, sluggish and hungry. That's when we reach for a "one-time-only" brownie or bag of potato chips. These high-G.I. foods deliver the rush we want and then let us down again. The roller-coaster ride is a hard cycle to break. But a high-G.I. diet will make you feel hungry more often, so you end up eating more and gaining more weight.

Let's look at the other end of the G.I. index. Low-G.I. foods, such as fruits, vegetables, whole grains, pasta, beans and low-fat dairy products, take longer to digest, deliver a steady supply of sugar to our bloodstream and leave us feeling fuller for a longer time. Consequently, we eat less. It also helps that these foods are lower in calories. As a result, we consume less food and fewer calories, without going hungry or feeling unsatisfied.

The key player in this process of energy storage and retrieval is insulin, a hormone secreted by the pancreas. Insulin does two things very well. First, it regulates the amount of sugar (glucose) in our bloodstream, removing the excess and storing it as glycogen for immediate use by our muscles, or putting it into storage as fat. Second, insulin acts as a security guard at the fat gates, reluctantly giving up its reserves. This evolutionary feature is a throwback to the days when our ancestors were hunter-gatherers, habitually experiencing times of feast or famine. When food was in abundance, the body stored its surplus as fat to tide it over the inevitable days of famine.

I was recently on vacation in a remote part of central Mexico, visiting the Copper Canyon, which, incredibly, is larger and deeper than the Grand Canyon in Arizona. A tribe of Tarahumara Indians still resides there. Until recently, these indigenous peoples typically put on thirty pounds during the summer and fall, when the crops, particularly corn, were plentiful. Then, over the course of the winter, when food became scarce, they lost these thirty pounds. Insulin was the champion in this process, both helping to accumulate fat and then guarding its depletion.

Of course, food is now readily available to us at the nearest twenty-four-hour supermarket. But our bodies still function very much as they did in the earliest days.

When we eat a high-G.I. food, our pancreas releases insulin to reduce the glucose level in our blood, which, if left unchecked, would lead to hyperglycemia. If we aren't using all that energy at the moment, the glucose is stored as fat. Soon we become hungry again. Our body can either draw on our reserves of fat and laboriously convert them back to sugar or it can look for more food. Since giving up extra fat is the body's last choice—who knows when that supply might come in handy!—our body would rather send us to the fridge than work to convert fat back to sugar. This helped serve survival back in the old days, but it gets in the way of weight loss now.

So our goal is to limit the amount of insulin in our system by avoiding high-G.I. foods, which stimulate its production, and instead choosing low-G.I. foods, which keep the supply of sugar in our bloodstream consistent. Slow-release, low-G.I. carbohydrates help curb your appetite by leaving you feeling fuller for a longer period of time. When you combine them with lean protein and the best fats, which help slow the digestive process, you have the

Dear Rick,

I'm sure you receive lots of terrific feedback from people, but I just wanted to pass along news of my success to you, nonetheless. I'm thrilled with the results I've had so far. I began eating the G.I. way at the beginning of September. I feel so much better and as of October 22, had lost 14 pounds.

As a grade six teacher, I used to feel like I would hit a wall at about 1:30 or 2:00 every afternoon. But now that my blood sugar levels are more consistent, I feel fine throughout the afternoon, and always have a food bar handy in my desk in case I feel a little hungry. I guess the best thing is that I don't feel deprived or that I'm on a diet. Rather, I feel I'm just eating better.

Thanks so much!

Mary

magic combination that will allow you to lose weight without going hungry.

Translated into real food, what does this mean? Well, for dinner you could have a grilled chicken breast, boiled new potatoes, a side salad of romaine lettuce and red pepper, dressed with a bit of olive oil and lemon, and some asparagus if you feel like it. The trick is to stick with foods that have a low G.I., are low in fat and are low-ish in calories. This sounds—and is, in fact—quite complex. It might seem to you as though I'm breaking my promise of an easy weight-loss plan. But don't worry: I've done all the calculations, measurements and math for you, and sorted the foods you like to eat into one of three categories based on the colours of the traffic light. This easy-to-follow colour-coded system means you will never have to count calories or points, or weigh and measure food. The G.I. Diet's emphasis on fruits and vegetables, whole grains, low-fat dairy products, lean protein and the "best" fats is a nutritionally ideal way to eat and doesn't eliminate any food groups. It will keep you feeling satisfied and energetic as you slim down to your ideal weight.

Now let's get into the details: what to eat, how much and how often.

What Do I Eat?

To find out what to eat and what to avoid to start losing weight, check out the Complete G.I. Diet Food Guide on pages 284–94. Here's how the colour-coded categories work:

Red-Light Foods
The foods in the red column are to be avoided. They are high-G.I., higher-calorie foods and are therefore red-light.

Yellow-Light Foods
The foods in the yellow column are mid-range G.I. foods and should be treated with caution. There are two phases in the G.I. Diet: Phase I is the weight-loss portion of the diet, and yellow-light foods should be avoided during this

time. Once you've reached your target weight, you enter Phase II, maintenance, and you can begin to enjoy yellow-light foods from time to time.

Green-Light Foods

The green column lists foods that are low-G.I., low in fat and lower in calories. These are the foods that will make you lose weight. Don't expect them to be tasteless and boring! There are many delicious and satisfying choices that will make you feel as though you aren't even on a diet.

If you're a veteran of the low-carbohydrate craze, you'll be surprised to find potatoes and rice in the green-light column, but they are fine as long as they are the right type. Baked potatoes and french fries have a high G.I., while boiled, small new potatoes have a low G.I. With rice, the short-grain, glutinous variety served in Chinese and Thai restaurants is high-G.I., while long-grain, brown, basmati and wild rice are low. Pasta is also a green-light food—as long as it is cooked only until al dente (with some firmness to the bite). Any processing of food, including cooking, will increase its G.I, since heat breaks down a food's starch capsules and fibre, giving your digestive juices a head start. This is why you should never overcook vegetables; instead steam them or boil them in a small amount of water just until they are tender. This way they will retain their vitamins and other nutrients, and their G.I. rating will remain low.

Chapter four outlines the best green-light options for breakfast, lunch, dinner and snacks.

How Much Do I Eat?

While following the G.I. program, you should be eating three meals and three snacks daily. Don't leave your digestive system with nothing to do. If your digestive system is busy processing food and steadily supplying energy to your brain, you won't be looking for high-calorie snacks.

You can, but for a few exceptions that I outline below, eat as much of the green-light foods as you like—within reason (five heads of cabbage is a bit extreme).

Green-Light Servings

Avocado	¼ of the fruit
Crispbreads (with high fibre, e.g., Wasa Fibre)	2 crispbreads
Green-light breads (which have at least 2½ to 3 grams of fibre per slice)	1 slice
Green-light cereals	½ cup
Green-light nuts	8 to 10
Margarine (nonhydrogenated, light)	2 teaspoons
Meat, fish, poultry	4 ounces (about the size of a pack of cards)
Olive/canola oil	1 teaspoon
Olives	4 to 5
Pasta	¾ cup cooked
Potatoes (new, boiled)	2 to 3
Rice (basmati, brown, long-grain)	⅔ cup cooked

PHASE II

Chocolate (at least 70 percent cocoa)	2 squares
Red wine	1 5-ounce glass

Portions

Each meal and snack should contain, if possible, a combination of green-light protein, carbohydrates—especially fruit and vegetables—and fats. An easy way to visualize portion size is to divide your plate into three sections (see illustration below). Half the plate should be filled with vegetables; one quarter should contain protein, such as lean meat, poultry, seafood, eggs, tofu or legumes; and the last quarter should contain a green-light serving of rice, pasta or potatoes.

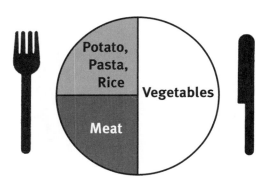

When Do I Eat?

Try to eat regularly throughout the day. If you skimp on breakfast and lunch, you will probably be starving by dinner and end up piling on the food. Have one snack mid-morning, another mid-afternoon and the last before bed.

The idea is to keep your digestive system happily busy so you won't start craving those red-light snacks.

Now that you know how the G.I. Diet works, it's time to get started. In the next chapter we'll outline the steps for launching you into Phase I.

Note: Before starting any major change in your eating patterns, make sure you check with your doctor.

TO SUM UP

- Low-G.I. foods take longer to digest, so you feel satiated longer.
- The key to losing weight is to eat low-G.I., low-calorie foods.
- In Phase I, eat only green-light foods.
- Eat three balanced meals and three snacks per day.
- Set aside a clothing allowance—you'll be needing new clothes!

CHAPTER THREE

Phase I: Reaching Your Target Weight

Phase I is the dramatic part of the G.I. Diet—the stage when those extra unwanted pounds come off! During this period you'll focus on eating green-light foods that are low-G.I. and also low in fat and sugar. Yes, this means a farewell to cheesecake and a fond adieu to bacon. But it doesn't mean you can't have the occasional fling. Falling off the wagon, while not encouraged, is acceptable as long as it's the exception and not the rule. This diet is not a straitjacket. If you do your best to eat the green-light way 90 percent of the time, you'll still lose weight. The odd lapse, at worst, will delay you by a week or two from reaching your target weight.

There are six steps in getting started on the green-light program. The first is to determine how much weight to lose.

1. Set your weight-loss target.

Since everyone has a distinct body type, metabolism and genes, there are no absolute rules for how much you should weigh. The only accepted international standard for weight is the Body Mass Index (BMI), a measurement of how much body fat you are carrying relative to your height.

You can calculate your BMI from the table on pages 34–35 by running your finger down the left vertical column of the table until you reach your height. Then run your finger across that row until you find the number that is closest to your weight. The bold number at the top of that column is your BMI.

If your BMI falls between 19 and 24, your weight is within the acceptable norm and is considered healthy. Anything between 25 and 29 is considered overweight; and if you're 30 or over, you are officially obese.

Too thin or too heavy is not good. Your health is at risk if your BMI falls below 18.5 or above 25. As a woman, with a lower muscle mass and smaller frame than most men, you might want to target the lower end of the healthy range, while men should generally target the higher end. However, if you are under eighteen, elderly or unusually muscle-bound—Serena Williams wouldn't fit on this chart—these ratings do not apply to you. For those over sixty-five, I suggest you allow yourself an extra 10 pounds to help protect you in case of a fall, or as an extra energy reserve if you get ill. Of course, this is only a guide, not an absolute. It is simply a good ballpark figure.

The other measurement you should concern yourself with is your waist measurement, which is an even better predictor of the state of your health than your weight. Abdominal fat is more than just a weight problem. Recent research has shown that abdominal fat acts almost like a separate organ in the body, except this "organ" is a destructive one that releases harmful proteins and free fatty acids into the rest of the body, increasing your risk of life-threatening conditions, especially heart disease.

If you are female and have a waist measurement of 35 inches or more, or male with a waist measurement of over 37 inches, you are at risk of endangering your health. Women with a measurement of 37 inches or more, and men with a measurement over 40 inches are at serious risk of heart disease, stroke, cancer and diabetes.

So I have your attention now! Make sure you measure correctly: put a tape measure around your waist at navel level till it fits snugly, without cutting into your flesh. Do not adopt the walking-down-the-beach-sucking-in-your-stomach stance. Just stand naturally. There's no point in trying to fudge the numbers, because the only person you're kidding is yourself.

Now that you know your BMI and waist measurement, you can set your weight loss target. On page 309, you will find a Weight/Waist Log for you to keep track of the pounds and inches you lose. There is nothing more motivating than recording your success, so be sure to weigh and measure yourself weekly and do it at the same time of day, since a meal or even a bowel movement can make a difference of a pound or two at a time when every pound counts! An ideal time is first thing in the morning, before breakfast.

Although I recommend recording your progress, please don't get obsessed with numbers on the scale. Many people find themselves losing inches before they register any weight loss on the scales. Clothes start feeling a little looser, and before you know it you are down a dress size or getting into your old jeans. Soon you'll probably have to buy new clothes. My readers often tell me that I should have warned them about the extra cost of refurbishing their closet!

Keep in mind that you will lose an average of one pound per week. I say average because most people do not lose weight at a fixed and steady rate. The usual pattern is to lose more at the start of the diet, when you are losing mostly water weight, followed by a series of drops and plateaus. The closer you get to your target weight, the slower your weight loss will be. If you are planning to lose up to 10 percent of your body weight—for example, if you weigh 150 pounds and want to lose 15 pounds—assume this will take you fifteen weeks, one pound per week. If you have more than 10 percent to shed, the good news is that you will lose at a faster rate. This is simply because your larger body requires more calories just to keep operating than someone who is lighter. Still, be prepared for measured, steady results—it took you a while to put on those extra pounds and it will take some time to lose them. Be patient and know that once that weight is gone, it will be gone forever as you keep it off in Phase II of the program.

			NORMAL					OVERWEIGHT				OBES
BMI	**19**	**20**	**21**	**22**	**23**	**24**	**25**	**26**	**27**	**28**	**29**	**30**	**31**
HEIGHT						WEIGHT	(POUNDS)					
4'10"	91	96	100	105	110	115	119	124	129	134	138	143	148
4'11"	94	99	104	109	114	119	124	128	133	138	143	148	153
5'0"	97	102	107	112	118	123	128	133	138	143	148	153	158
5'1"	100	106	111	116	122	127	132	137	143	148	153	158	164
5'2"	104	109	115	120	126	131	136	142	147	153	158	164	169
5'3"	107	113	118	124	130	135	141	146	152	158	163	169	175
5'4"	110	116	122	128	134	140	145	151	157	163	169	174	180
5'5"	114	120	126	132	138	144	150	156	162	168	174	180	186
5'6"	118	124	130	136	142	148	155	161	167	173	179	186	192
5'7"	121	127	134	140	146	153	159	166	172	178	185	191	198
5'8"	125	131	138	144	151	158	164	171	177	184	190	197	203
5'9"	128	135	142	149	155	162	169	176	182	189	196	203	209
5'10"	132	139	146	153	160	167	174	181	188	195	202	209	216
5'11"	136	143	150	157	165	172	179	186	193	200	208	215	222
6'0"	140	147	154	162	169	177	184	191	199	206	213	221	228
6'1"	144	151	159	166	174	182	189	197	204	212	219	227	235
6'2"	148	155	163	171	179	186	194	202	210	218	225	233	241
6'3"	152	160	168	176	184	192	200	208	216	224	232	240	248
6'4"	156	164	172	180	189	197	205	213	221	230	238	246	254

BODY MAS

Source: U.S. National Heart, Lung and Blood Institute

INDEX (BMI)

			OBESE					EXTREME OBESITY					
32	33	34	35	36	37	38	39	40	41	42	43	44	45
WEIGHT (POUNDS)													
153	158	162	167	172	177	181	186	191	196	201	205	210	215
158	163	168	173	178	183	188	193	198	203	208	212	217	222
163	168	174	179	184	189	194	199	204	209	215	220	225	230
169	174	180	185	190	195	201	206	211	217	222	227	232	238
175	180	186	191	196	202	207	213	218	224	229	235	240	246
180	186	191	197	203	208	214	220	225	231	237	242	248	254
186	192	197	204	209	215	221	227	232	238	244	250	256	262
192	198	204	210	216	222	228	234	240	246	252	258	264	270
198	204	210	216	223	229	235	241	247	253	260	266	272	278
204	211	217	223	230	236	242	249	255	261	268	274	280	287
210	216	223	230	236	243	249	256	262	269	276	282	289	295
216	223	230	236	243	250	257	263	270	277	284	291	297	304
222	229	236	243	250	257	264	271	278	285	292	299	306	313
229	236	243	250	257	265	272	279	286	293	301	308	315	322
235	242	250	258	265	272	279	287	294	302	309	316	324	331
242	250	257	265	272	280	288	295	302	310	318	325	333	340
249	256	264	272	280	287	295	303	311	319	326	334	342	350
256	264	272	279	287	295	303	311	319	327	335	343	351	359
263	271	279	287	295	304	312	320	328	336	344	353	361	369

2. Clear out the cupboards/ pantry/fridge.

Take a look in your fridge—what do you see? Two jars of mayonnaise, some leftover Cheddar and a lot of sugar-laden condiments in jars? Now open the cupboards: what's the cookie and cracker situation? Now is the time to do an honest evaluation of what you tend to keep on hand. Consult the Complete G.I. Diet Food Guide (pages 284–94) and throw out anything that's in the red-light column. Be ruthless. If you always have chips on hand, let's face it—you will eat them. If you keep Goldfish crackers around "for the kids," you can be sure that they won't be the only ones snacking on them. If you hate waste, give the unopened food items and cans to your skinny neighbours or local food bank. When you banish red-light foods from your house, it will be a clear sign to your family that you're serious about eating the healthier, G.I. way. (Tips on getting your spouse and children on-board can be found in Part II: The Family.)

3. Eat before you shop.

You know what happens when you drop by the supermarket on your way home from work, famished—before you know it you've bought the biggest tray of cannelloni ever made. The worst mistake you can make it is to go shopping on an empty stomach. You'll only be tempted to fill your cart with high-G.I., sugar-rich foods.

4. Shop green-light.

Consult chapter four to get some ideas of what you'd like to have for breakfast, lunch, dinner and snacks during your first week on the G.I. Diet. Peruse the recipe section in part three and look at the Complete G.I. Diet Food Guide on pages 284–94. (You could also pick up a copy of *The G.I. Diet Guide to Shopping and Eating Out*.) Write out a shopping list and head out to the supermarket. Your first few green-light shopping trips will require a bit more time and attention than usual, as you familiarize yourself with green-light eating and meal planning. But don't worry, before long your new shopping and eating habits will become second nature.

Since it would be impossible to include every brand available in today's enormous supermarkets in the G.I. Diet Food Guide, I've listed categories of food rather than individual brands, except in cases where clarification is needed, or there is an especially useful product available. This means that you will have to pay some attention to food labels. Some brands of the foods I list in the green-light column may contain red-light ingredients, like sugar or trans fatty acids.

When reading a food label, there are five factors to consider when making the best green-light choice:

Serving Size

Is the serving size realistic, or has the manufacturer lowered it so the calories and fat levels look better than the competition's? When comparing one brand with another, make sure you are comparing the same serving size.

Nutrition Facts
Valeur nutritive
Serving 1 cup (55 g)
Portion de 1 tasse (55 g)

| Amount Per Serving | % Daily Value |
| Teneur par portion | % valeur quotidienne |

Calories / Calories 190	
Fat / Lipides 1.5 g	**2** %
Saturated / saturés 0 g	**0** %
+ Trans / trans 0 g	
Cholesterol / Cholestérol 0 mg	**0** %
Sodium / Sodium 90 mg	**4** %
Potassium / Potassium 500 mg	**14** %
Carbohydrate / Glucides 31 g	**10** %
Fibre / Fibres 10 g	**42** %
Sugars / Sucres 6 g	
Protein / Protéines 14 g	
Vitamin A / Vitamine A	0 %
Vitamin C / Vitamine C	0 %
Calcium / Calcium	6 %
Iron / Fer	15 %
Phosphorus / Phosphore	20 %

Calories

The product with the least amount of calories is obviously the best choice. Sometimes products flagged as "low-fat" still have plenty of calories, so don't be fooled by the diet-friendly slogans. Calories are calories, whether they come from fat or sugar.

Fat

Look at the amount of fat, which is often expressed as a percentage, say 2 percent (good) or 20 percent (forget it). Then check to see what sort of fat it is. You want foods that are low-fat, with minimal or no saturated fats and trans fats. Remember that trans fats are often called "hydrogenated oils" or "partially hydrogenated oils."

Fibre

Foods with lots of fibre have a low G.I., so this is an important component. When comparing brands, choose the one with higher fibre.

Sugar

Choose products that are low in sugar. Again, watch for products advertised as "low-fat." Sometimes companies will quietly bump up the sugar content to make up for any perceived loss of taste. This often happens with yogurts and cereals.

Dear Rick,

My family doctor informed me about your book and put me on your diet. After many years of trying many diets, diet groups, etc., I was never very successful. I may have lost a few pounds, but was not able to keep it off. On the G.I. Diet, I have lost 22 pounds and want to lose another 15. I find the program extremely easy to follow—it has become a way of life for me now. I like the way I feel—in control—the way I look, and the confidence I now have. I'm determined to reach my target weight and show my friends and family the new me! My doctor says I'm his star patient.

Thank you, thank you!

Sincerely, Bobbi

Sugars are sometimes listed as dextrose, glucose, fructose or sucrose—regardless of the form, it's sugar.

Sodium

Sodium (salt) increases water retention, which doesn't help when you are trying to lose weight. It also contributes to premenstrual bloating in women and is a factor in hypertension (high blood pressure). Combine high blood pressure with excess weight and you move up to the front of the risk line for heart disease and stroke. Low-sodium products are therefore preferable.

The Recommended Daily Allowance (RDA) for sodium is 2,500 mg, but this is generally regarded as too high. The U.S. National Academy of Science's new recommendation of 1,500 mg makes more sense. Since the average North American consumption of sodium per person per day is over 3,000 mg, it goes without saying that most of us could stand to cut back. However, if you have a BMI of over 30 and have any blood pressure, circulation or heart problems, you need to be even more vigilant about seeking out low-sodium brands. Canned foods like soups are often very high in sodium, as are many fast foods.

5. Eat the green-light way.

You've cracked the label codes and restocked your pantry. Now all you have to do on Phase I is eat three green-light meals and three green-light snacks each day and you're on your way to your new trim self. You will soon begin to feel better and your cravings will stop. It won't be long before you reach your target weight.

6. Exercise.

Diet has far more impact on weight loss than exercise does. You can spend an hour on the treadmill and expend only 250 calories, which you can put right back on again if you eat half a large muffin on the way home. The following chart shows the amount of effort required to lose just one pound of fat.

	EFFORT REQUIRED TO LOSE 1 LB OF FAT	
	130-lb person	160-lb person
Walking (4 mph–brisk)	53 miles/85 km	42 miles/67 km
Running (8 min/mile)	36 miles/58 km	29 miles/46 km
Cycling (12–14 mph)	96 miles/154 km	79 miles/127 km
Sex (moderate effort)	79 times	64 times

Not many of us are going to cycle 96 miles just to lose a pound, and while making love seventy-nine times might sound like a pleasant way to lose a pound, this would definitely cut into your schedule! Still, regular, moderate exercise is very important in the long term, both for maintaining your new weight and for staying healthy. For example, if you were to walk briskly for half an hour a day, seven days a week, you would burn up calories equalling 20 pounds of fat per year. This means that in Phase I, exercise is not essential to your weight-loss program, but it is an important consideration in Phase II, where you maintain your new weight. As well, for women past menopause, weight-bearing exercise is one way to counteract osteoporosis and the risk of fractures. And for families, exercising together— biking, skiing, whatever you enjoy—not only helps control weight but is also a way to enjoy each other's company.

Before you start shedding pounds, it might be hard to get out there and hit the gym or walk. But once you lose a bit of weight, being active will be something you enjoy and actually look forward to. So stick with it—the fun will kick in eventually.

Before we go any further, we should define exactly what we mean by exercise. There are three basic types of exercise, each working in a synergistic relationship with the others.

Aerobic

The objective of aerobic exercise is to get your heart and lungs working harder. Aerobic exercise, such as walking, jogging, biking, swimming, hiking and so on, will have the most impact on your overall weight and health. In chapter eleven, there is more discussion about the impact of weight on your health, particularly heart disease, stroke and diabetes, which account for five deaths out of every ten.

Strength

Strength training is particularly important as we move into middle age and beyond because of the steady reduction in muscle mass that accompanies aging. Starting at the age of twenty-five, the body loses 2 percent of its muscle mass each decade, a process that accelerates to 6 to 8 percent as we move into our senior years.

By exercising muscles on a regular basis, the loss can be minimized or reversed. And why is that important? Because the larger your muscles, the more energy (calories) they use. When you're at rest, or even asleep in bed, your muscles are using energy. So keeping or building muscle mass really helps you burn calories and lose weight.

Though regular exercise will help minimize muscle loss, it is through resistance exercises that we actually build muscle mass. Resistance exercises involve fixed or free weights, elastic bands or even your own body weight; pushing your hands together as hard as you can is a form of resistance exercise. You don't have to join a gym and work out with massive barbells. A few simple exercises, easily done at home, will do wonders to tone and restore those flabby muscles.

At the same time, strength training consumes calories. So whether at work or at rest, increased muscle mass helps you lose or maintain your weight.

Stretching

Again this is a significant issue as we age and lose flexibility in our joints, tendons and ligaments. Loss of flexibility reduces our ability to do either aerobic or strength training, both of which depend on healthy joints and tissues. In older people, this loss of flexibility can lead to falls and hip fractures. So although stretching may seem like a "frill," it is central to the whole fitness picture.

Stretching exercises will also give you the biggest bang for your buck in terms of immediate payout. Within just a week, you can increase your flexibility by over 100 percent. Both aerobic and strength training can actually make you less flexible if you don't stretch those muscle ligaments and tendons. That's why you always see athletes warming up and down with stretching exercises. So always include stretching, whether a simple set of muscle stretches or a yoga or Tai Chi session, in your exercise program. (See page 51.)

Now let's review your options.

Outdoor Activities

Walking

This is by far the simplest and, for most people, the easiest exercise program to start and maintain. For adults, thirty minutes a day, seven days a week, should be your target. If you add an hour-long walk on the weekend, you can take a day off during the week. As mentioned before, we're talking about brisk walking, not speed walking nor ambling along. Imagine you're late for an appointment. The pace should increase your heart and breathing rates, but never to the point where you lack the breath to talk with a partner.

You don't need any special clothing or equipment, except a pair of comfortable cushioned shoes or sneakers. And walking is rarely boring since you can keep changing routes and watch the world go by. Walk with an older son or daughter for company and mutual support, or go solo and commune with nature and your own thoughts. If you have a child in a stroller, you can set a brisk pace that way, or invest in a jogger stroller. I prefer to walk on my own in the morning, which is when I do my best thinking of the day. This is not surprising when you realize how much extra oxygen-fresh blood is pumping through the brain.

A great idea for working people is to incorporate walking into the daily commute. I used to get off the bus three stops early on my way to and from work. Those three stops are equal to about one and a half miles, so I was walking about three miles per day! If you drive to work, try parking your car about one and a half miles away and walk to your job. You may even find cheaper parking farther away. However, start with just one stop early and work yourself up. Who knows—distance permitting, you may eventually be able to walk to work. Think of the savings in gas and parking fees!

Jogging

This is similar to walking, but you need the proper
footwear to protect joints from damage. The advantage of
jogging over walking is that it approximately doubles the
number of calories burned in the same period of time:
400 calories for jogging versus 200 for brisk walking over
a thirty-minute period. While walking, try jogging for a
few yards and see if this is for you. Jogging gets your heart
rate up, which is great for heart health. The heart is basically a muscle and, like all muscles, it thrives on being
exercised, so in general, the more the better. If jogging
suits you, then this could be the simplest and most effective method of exercise as it uses personal time efficiently,
can be done anytime, anywhere, and is inexpensive.

Hiking

Another variation on walking is cross-country hiking.
Because this usually involves different kinds of terrain,
especially hills and valleys, you use up more calories,
about 50 percent more than for brisk walking. The reason
for this is that you expend considerably more energy going
uphill. Try hauling 150 to 200 pounds up a hill and you'll
get some idea of the extra effort your body has to make.

Hiking is fun, too, and is an especially good motivator
for the whole family. It's an excuse for a special excursion
out of town and for some adventure that can include every
age, even a baby in a backpack. The only caveat is to
choose a route that offers a variety of loops, from short to
long. If your younger children flag, you can make your

hikes suitable to the limits of the smallest. One way to satisfy everyone's level of fitness is to take turns: while you are with the "slow pack"—one parent plus the kids—your partner jogs or walks ahead, then loops back to join you and trade. This gives everyone a satisfying outing.

Bicycling

Like walking, jogging and hiking, bicycling is a fun way to burn up calories, and it is almost as effective as jogging. For people with low-back or knee problems, it can be preferable. Other than the cost of the bike, it's inexpensive and can be done almost anywhere, anytime, with helmets, plus lights and reflectors for night riding, of course.

Sports

Although most sports are terrific calorie burners, they usually cannot be part of a regular routine. Most of them require other people, equipment and facilities. But they can provide a boost to your regular fitness and exercise program. Such popular sports as tennis, basketball, soccer, softball and golf (no golf cart, please) are excellent additions to a basic exercise program. However, they're no substitute for a five- to seven-day-a-week regular schedule.

Indoor Activities

Many of you will be muttering by now about how this would all be fine advice if we lived in California. But many of us must contend with either frigid, snowy winters or hot, humid summers, which limit outdoor activities.

The alternatives are either to organize a home gym or join a fitness club. The advantage of clubs is that they offer a wide range of sophisticated equipment, with instruction and advice from staff. Clubs are also social, and some people find they need group motivation to work out with enthusiasm. YMCAs also offer special programs for the elderly, new mothers and those with special needs, and some provide subsidies for people who can't afford the membership fees. Many community centres offer free fitness classes, too.

If a fitness club isn't convenient or those Lycra-clad young things make you uncomfortable, you can always set up your exercise area at home. The best and least expensive piece of equipment is a stationary bike. The latest models work on magnetic resistance rather than the old friction strap around the flywheel. This gives a smoother action, with better tension adjustment. Most important, they are quiet, which is crucial if you want to be able to listen to music or watch TV.

You can easily pay in the thousands for a bike with all the fancy trimmings, but the $250 to $300 machines will work fine. Just be sure you choose one that has smooth, adjustable tension; then, pop in that late-night movie or your favourite soap and get pedalling. You'll be amazed how quickly the minutes fly by. Twenty minutes on the bike consumes the same number of calories as thirty minutes of brisk walking.

If biking is not for you, try a treadmill. These can be

expensive, and beware of the lower-end models that cannot take the pounding. Expect to pay about $1,000 and up. Make sure the incline of the track can be raised and lowered for a better workout. Both treadmills and bikes can simulate outdoor walking, jogging, hiking or biking in the comfort of your own home. I use both of these machines but have added a cross-country ski machine, which has the advantage of working the upper body as well. Ski machines are generally less expensive than treadmills, but they cost more than stationary bikes. They also burn a higher number of calories (similar to jogging) because they use the arms and shoulders as well as the legs. It's almost the perfect all-body workout machine.

There are several other specialized options, such as stair climber machines, elliptical walkers and rowing machines, but they're not for everyone. They are also quite expensive, so make sure you try them out first at a fitness club or with a cooperative retailer.

Strength Training

It's now time to pay some attention to rebuilding your muscle mass. Remember that after age forty, you will lose between four and six pounds of muscle every decade, which is usually replaced with flab. That's four to six pounds of calorie-consuming muscle. Muscles burn up energy even when idle. Bigger muscles consume more energy than smaller muscles. So muscles come in handy for losing weight.

Resistance-training equipment can range from the complex and expensive to a $10 rubber band. Home gyms, with prices that begin at a couple hundred dollars, are a popular option. For most people, however, there are cheaper, simpler methods, such as a set of free weights or (my own preference) rubber exercise bands. Dyna-Band and Thera-Band are two popular choices. I like using Thera-Bands, which come in varying thicknesses that offer increasing levels of resistance as you regain and build your muscle strength.

These resistance rubber bands and weights are available at many fitness exercise equipment retailers and surgical supply stores. Try a few resistance exercises, concentrating on the larger muscle groups—your legs, arms and upper chest. These are the muscles that will give you the biggest bang by burning up the most calories. The resistance exercises should complement your other regular exercise regimen, not replace it. Committing to both types of exercise will produce far better results than either one alone. And resistance exercises are best done every other day, leaving time for your muscles to recuperate.

Pilates

I've recently become a Pilates enthusiast. Originally, it was recommended by my physiotherapist to strengthen my back and prevent my disc problem from recurring. However, this very precise system of exercises does a lot more than just that. It's a series of floor exercises—no equipment needed—that both strengthen and stretch your muscles, especially the core muscles in your back and around your waist, which are essential for good posture. It's great for any level of fitness and at any age, and it is much less boring than step classes or other gym routines.

Yoga and Tai Chi

Yoga comes in different styles now: hatha, kundalini, kripalu, ashtanga, bikram and others. If you're new to yoga, the best choice is hatha, which teaches you simple postures that will keep you supple, offer relaxation techniques and improve your breathing and circulation. Ashtanga is trendy nowadays, but it is more aerobic and demanding. Kundalini focuses more on energizing breathing techniques and meditation. But in any form, this ancient practice has much to offer, especially to anyone taking up exercise in middle age.

Tai Chi is another Eastern discipline that is gentle, promoting flexibility, balance and energy. It features a series of flowing postures, done standing, that many people like to practise early in the morning, out of doors. It keeps the joints and tendons supple, and offers a peaceful, revitalizing form of activity that can carry you into old age. With both Tai Chi and yoga, there are a number of instructional DVDs or videos available for those who want to learn or practise at home.

As this is a book on nutrition, not exercise, I have not included any exercises for either stretching or strength training, particularly as there are a great number of excellent books on the subject. Check your local bookstore. Or you can consult the web for free. The U.S. government website is a gold mine, so you can always start there: www.niapublications.org/exercisebook/exercisebook.asp. For suggestions about incorporating physical activity into your daily life, check out the Canadian Public Health Agency website, at www.phac-aspc.gc.ca/pau-uap/fitness.

Follow these six steps and you will be well on your way to reaching your weight-loss target. Remember not to despair if you fall off the wagon now and then. The mistake many people make is too feel so bad about one wrong move that they give up. Don't be so hard on yourself! If you're living on the program 90 percent of the time, you will still successfully lose.

TO SUM UP
The five steps to get you launched in Phase I are:
1. Set your weight/waist goal.
2. Clear the decks: pantry, fridge and freezer.
3. Go green-light shopping and read your labels.
4. Eat the green-light way.
5. Include some exercise in your daily routine.

CHAPTER FOUR

Meal Basics

Because the green-light way of eating is most likely new to you, you're probably wondering what to eat instead of that bagel with cream cheese for breakfast, that hamburger for lunch, and those tortilla chips and salsa for a snack. Well this chapter specifically outlines what you can and cannot eat for the three main meals and snacks that are part of your daily G.I. program. Let's start with breakfast.

Breakfast

I know you've been told that breakfast is the most important meal of the day—well, it's true. It's the first thing you eat after your night-long "fast" of twelve hours or more, and it launches you into your workday. Eating a healthy breakfast will help you avoid the need to grab a coffee and Danish as soon as you hit the office, and will make you feel satisfied and energetic. Eating breakfast every day doesn't mean you have to set the alarm any earlier. If you have time to read the paper or feed the cat, you have time to prepare and eat a green-light breakfast.

The following chart lists typical breakfast foods in the colour-coded categories. To ensure you have a balanced breakfast, include some green-light carbohydrates, protein and fat. For a complete list of foods, see the Complete G.I. Diet Food Guide on pages 284–94.

PROTEIN			
Meat and Eggs	Regular bacon Sausages Whole regular eggs	Turkey bacon Whole omega-3 eggs	Back bacon Lean ham Liquid eggs/egg whites
Dairy	Cheese Cottage cheese (whole or 2%) Cream Milk (whole or 2%) Sour cream Yogurt (whole or 2%)	Cream cheese (light) Milk (1%) Sour cream (light) Yogurt (low-fat with sugar)	Buttermilk Cheese (fat-free) Cottage cheese (1% or fat-free) Fruit yogurt (non-fat with sugar substitute) Milk (skim) Soy milk (plain, low-fat)
CARBOHYDRATES			
Cereals	All cold cereals except those listed as yellow- or green-light Granola Muesli (commercial)	Kashi Go Lean Crunch Kashi Good Friends Red River Shredded Wheat Bran	All-Bran Bran Buds Fibre First Kashi Go Lean Oat Bran Porridge (old-fashioned rolled oats)

Breads/ Grains	Bagels Baguette Cookies Doughnuts Muffins Pancakes/Waffles White bread	Crispbreads (with fibre) Whole grain breads*	100% stone-ground whole wheat* Crispbreads (high fibre, e.g., Wasa Fibre)* Green-light muffins (see pp. 274–77) Whole-grain, high-fibre breads (2½-3g fibre per slice)*
Fruits	Applesauce containing sugar Canned fruit in syrup Melons Most dried fruit	Apricots ** (fresh and dried) Bananas Dried cranberries** Fruit cocktail in juice Kiwi Mango Papaya Pineapple	Apples Berries Cherries Grapefruit Grapes Oranges Peaches Plums
Juices	Fruit drinks Prune Sweetened juices Watermelon	Apple (unsweetened) Grapefruit (unsweetened) Orange (unsweetened) Pear (unsweetened)	Eat the fruit rather than drink its juice
Vege- tables	French fries Hash browns		Most vegetables

* Limit serving size (see page 27).
** For baking, it is OK to use a modest amount of dried apricots or cranberries.

FATS		
Butter	Most nuts	Almonds*
Hard margarine	Natural nut butters	Canola oil*
Peanut butter (regular and light)	Natural peanut butter	Hazelnuts*
Tropical oils	Soft margarine (non-hydrogenated)	Olive oil*
Vegetable shortening	Vegetable oils	Soft margarine (non-hydrogenated, light)*

* Limit serving size (see page 27).

Let's take a closer look at some of the usual breakfast choices.

Coffee and Tea

OK, this is the toughest one. The trouble with coffee is caffeine. It's not a health problem in itself, but it does stimulate the production of insulin. That's part of the "buzz" we get from coffee. But insulin reduces blood sugar levels, which then increases your appetite. Have you ever ordered a Venti from Starbucks and then felt positively shaky an hour later? That's your blood sugar hitting bottom. You cure it by eating a bagel—which isn't helpful when you're trying to lose weight. So in Phase I, try to cut out caffeine altogether. As unpleasant as it may be, caffeine withdrawal will end in a day or two. Cut down gradually: go from a medium coffee to a small; then try a half-caffeinated, half-decaf blend. Then limit yourself to decaffeinated coffee—some brands taste as good as the real thing.

Even better, switch to tea. It has only about a third of the caffeine that coffee has, and black tea has health benefits as well: it's rich in antioxidants, and beneficial for heart health and reducing the risk of dementias. Green tea is also considered an anti-carcinogen. (My ninety-five-year-old mother and her tea-drinking cronies are living proof!) Herbal teas, such as peppermint, chamomile and other blends, are fine too, as long as they contain no caffeine.

If no coffee is going to be a deal breaker, then go ahead, have one cup a day—but not a double espresso. If you take milk and sugar, make it skim milk and a sweetener such as Splenda.

Cereals

Another toughie. Most cold cereals contain hidden or not-so-hidden sugars, and are therefore red-light. Green-light cereals are high in fibre; they have at least 10 grams per serving. All right, they're not a lot of fun by themselves, but you can liven them up with fresh, canned or frozen fruits, a few nuts and some fruit yogurt (fat-free, with sugar substitute).

My personal favourite cereal is good old-fashioned oatmeal—not the instant type that comes in packets but the large-flake, slow-cooking kind. (They're starting to serve it in the smartest hotels now.) Not only is large-flake oatmeal low-G.I., but it's also low-calorie and has been shown to lower cholesterol. Yes, you have to cook it, but it only takes about three minutes or so in the microwave, and not much longer for one portion on the stovetop. Dress it up with yogurt, sliced almonds, berries or unsweetened applesauce. It's also just fine with nothing but milk on it.

I probably receive more emails about people's delight in rediscovering oatmeal than about any other food or meal. Give it a try.

Toast

Go ahead, but have no more than one slice per meal. Make sure your bread has at least 2.5 to 3 grams of fibre per slice. (Note: Most bread labels quote a two-slice serving, which should equal 5 to 6 grams per serving.) The best choice is 100% stone-ground whole wheat bread, which has a coarser grind and therefore a lower G.I. White bread, cracked wheat or anything else made with white flour is red-light.

Butter and Jams

Butter is out. It's very high in saturated fat, and despite the protestations of the dairy industry, it's not good for your health or waistline. Yes, it does make things taste good—that's what fat does best. But you can still enjoy any one of a variety of light non-hydrogenated soft margarines, if you use only a teaspoon or so.

When buying fruit spreads, look for the "extra fruit/no sugar added" varieties. Fruit, not sugar, should be the first ingredient listed. They taste great and don't have the calories of the usual commercial jams. Although I rarely plug brands, the President's Choice Blue Menu jams are a good buy.

Dairy

Low-fat dairy products are an ideal green-light choice and an excellent source of protein. I have a glass of skim milk every morning. I admit that skim didn't taste great at first, but I weaned myself off 2% by switching to 1% before moving on to skim. Now 2% tastes like cream!

Fat-free yogurt with sugar substitute instead of sugar is ideal for breakfast, dessert or a snack, either by itself or added to fruits or cereals. Low-fat cottage cheese is also a top-rated green-light source of protein. Or you can make a low-fat soft cheese spread by letting yogurt drain in cheesecloth overnight in the refrigerator.

Regular, full-fat dairy products, including whole milk and cream, cheese and butter are loaded with saturated fat and should be avoided completely.

Eggs

Use liquid eggs, such as Naturegg Break Free or Omega Pro. They are lower in saturated fat and cholesterol than regular eggs, and they make wonderful omelettes. Otherwise, use egg whites. If you're eating a hotel breakfast, in most cases the kitchen is happy to make omelettes with egg whites only.

Bacon

Bacon is red-light because of its high saturated fat content. However, there are tasty green-light alternatives, such as Canadian back bacon, turkey bacon and lean ham—which make great BLTs.

Lunch

Lunch is usually the most problematic meal for my readers because they tend to eat it outside the home and in a hurry. However, with a little strategizing you'll have no problem eating green-light. You have two options: brown bag your lunch, packing items from your green-light pantry, or eat out at a restaurant or fast-food outlet. Here are the ground rules. For a complete list of foods, see the Complete G.I. Diet Food Guide on pages 284–94.

PROTEIN			
Meat, Poultry, Fish and Eggs	Ground beef (more than 10% fat)	Ground beef (lean)	All fish and seafood, fresh or frozen (no batter or breading) or canned
	Hamburgers	Lamb (lean cuts)	
	Hot dogs	Pork (lean cuts)	
	Pâté	Turkey bacon	Beef (lean cuts)
	Processed meats	Whole omega-3 eggs	Chicken/Turkey breast (skinless)
	Regular bacon	Tofu	Ground beef (extra-lean)
	Sausages		Lean deli ham
	Whole regular eggs		Liquid eggs (e.g., Break Free)
			Tofu (low-fat)
			Veal
Dairy	Cheese	Milk (1%)	Cheese (fat-free)
	Cottage cheese (whole or 2%)	Cheese (low-fat)	Cottage cheese (1% or fat-free)
	Cream cheese	Yogurt (low-fat with sugar)	Fruit yogurt (non-fat with sugar substitute)
	Milk (whole or 2%)	Cream cheese (light)	Ice cream (low-fat and no added sugar)
			Milk (skim)

CARBOHYDRATES

Breads/ Grains	Bagels		Crispbreads (with fibre, e.g. Ryvita High Fibre)	100% stone-ground whole wheat bread*
	Baguette/ Croissants			
	Croutons		Pita (whole wheat)	Crispbreads (high fibre, e.g., Wasa Fibre)
	Cake/Cookies		Tortillas (whole wheat)	
	Hamburger/ Hotdog buns		Whole grain breads*	Pasta* (fettuccine, spaghetti, penne, vermicelli, linguine, macaroni)
	Macaroni and cheese			
	Muffins/Doughnuts			Quinoa
	Noodles (canned or instant)			Rice (basmati, wild, brown, long-grain)
	Pancakes/Waffles			Whole-grain, high-fibre breads ($2\frac{1}{2}$–3 g fibre per slice)*
	Pasta filled with cheese or meat			
	Pizza			
	Rice (short grain, white, instant)			

Fruits/ Vege- tables	Broad beans	Apricots	Apples	Carrots
	French fries	Artichokes	Arugula	Cauliflower
	Melons	Bananas	Asparagus	Celery
	Most dried fruit	Beets	Avocado*	Cherries
		Corn	Beans (green/wax)	Cucumbers
	Parsnips	Kiwi		Eggplant
	Potatoes (mashed or baked)	Mangoes	Bell peppers	Grapefruit
		Papaya	Blackberries	Grapes
	Rutabaga	Pineapple	Broccoli	Leeks
		Potatoes (boiled)	Brussels sprouts	Lemons
		Squash	Cabbage	Lettuce

* Limit serving size (see page 27).

Sweet potatoes	Mushrooms	Plums
Yams	Olives*	Potatoes (boiled new)
	Onions	Radishes
	Oranges (all varieties)	Raspberries
	Peaches	Snow peas
	Pears	Spinach
	Peas	Strawberries
	Peppers (hot)	Tomatoes
	Pickles	Zucchini

FATS

Butter	Mayonnaise (light)	Almonds*
Hard margarine	Most nuts	Canola oil*
Mayonnaise	Natural peanut butter (no added sugar)	Mayonnaise (fat-free)
Peanut butter (regular, light)	Salad dressings (light)	Olive oil*
Salad dressings (regular)	Soft margarine (non-hydrogenated)	Salad dressings (low-fat, low sugar)
Tropical oils		Soft margarine (non-hydrogenated, light)

SOUPS

All cream-based soups	Canned chicken noodle	Chunky bean and vegetable soups (e.g., Campbell's Healthy Request, Healthy Choice, and Too Good To Be True)
Canned black bean	Canned lentil	
Canned green pea	Canned tomato	
Canned puréed vegetable		
Canned split pea		

* Limit serving size (see page 27).

The Brown Bag Option

Bringing your own lunch to work is the easiest way to ensure you eat green-light. And if you're a mother or father who already has to pack school lunches, all you have to do is assemble one more, for you. There are other advantages to brown-bagging it, besides avoiding the temptation of a red-light lunch: it's cheaper, and it gives you downtime at your desk to read or catch up on paperwork.

Sandwiches

Sandwiches are the lunchtime staple, and it's no wonder: they're portable, easy to make and offer endless variety. They can also be a dietary disaster, but if you follow the suggestions below, you can keep your sandwiches green-light.

- Always use 100% stone-ground whole wheat or high-fibre whole grain bread (2 ½ to 3 grams of fibre per slice).
- Sandwiches should be served open-faced. Either pack components separately and assemble just before eating or make your sandwich with a "lettuce lining" that helps keep the bread from getting soggy.
- Include at least three vegetables, such as lettuce, tomato, red or green bell pepper, cucumber, sprouts or onion.
- Instead of spreading the bread with butter or margarine, use mustard or hummus.
- Add up to 4 ounces of cooked lean meat or fish: roast beef, turkey, shrimp or salmon.

- If you make tuna or chicken salad, use low-fat mayonnaise or low-fat salad dressing and celery.
- Mix canned salmon with malt vinegar or fresh lemon.

Salads

Preparing salads may seem more labour-intensive than sandwiches, but it doesn't have to be. Invest in a variety of reusable plastic containers so you can bring individual-sized salads to work. Keep a supply of green-light vinaigrette on hand, and wash greens ahead of time and store in paper towels in plastic bags. You'll find that salads are a creative way to use up leftovers with a minimum of fuss.

Basic Salad

1 ½ cups	lettuce (such as romaine, leaf, Boston, iceberg, mesclun, arugula, watercress or baby spinach), torn or coarsely chopped
1	small carrot, grated
½	red, yellow or green bell pepper, diced
1	plum tomato, cut into wedges
½ cup	sliced cucumber
¼ cup	chopped red onion (optional)
	Basic Green-Light Vinaigrette (recipe follows)

In bowl, toss together lettuce, carrot, bell pepper, tomato, cucumber and onion. Pour vinaigrette over greens and toss.

Makes 1 serving.

Variations: To make a meal out of this salad, add some protein with 4 oz canned tuna, cooked salmon, tofu, kidney beans, chickpeas, cooked chicken or another lean meat.

Instead of making Basic Green-Light Vinaigrette, you can use the same amount of a low-fat, low-sugar, store-bought dressing.

Basic Green-Light Vinaigrette

1 tbsp	vinegar (such as white, red wine, balsamic, rice or cider, or you can use lemon juice)
1 tsp	extra-virgin olive oil or canola oil
½ tsp	Dijon mustard
1	clove garlic, crushed (optional)
Pinch	each salt and black pepper
Pinch	dried or fresh herb of choice (such as thyme, oregano, basil, marjoram, mint or Italian seasoning)

In small bowl, whisk together vinegar, oil, mustard, garlic, salt, pepper and herbs.

Makes 1 serving.

Storage: Both the salad and the dressing can be prepared ahead and stored separately, covered, for about two days.

Salade Niçoise

2	small new potatoes, skins on, cooked and quartered
1 cup	green beans, cooked
1 cup	torn or coarsely chopped lettuce
1 tbsp	Basic Green-Light Vinaigrette, or other low-fat dressing
2 oz	canned tuna, drained and flaked
1	hard-boiled omega-3 egg, peeled and quartered
1	medium tomato, quartered
1	anchovy fillet (optional)
6	pitted black olives
	Chopped fresh parsley
	Salt and black pepper

In serving bowl, combine potatoes, beans and lettuce. Add vinaigrette and toss gently. Place tuna in centre and arrange wedges of egg and tomato around it. Add the anchovy, if using, and sprinkle with olives and parsley. Season with salt and pepper to taste.

Makes 1 serving.

Fresh Fish Option: Substitute grilled fresh tuna or other fish for the canned tuna.

Waldorf Chicken and Rice Salad

1 cup	cooked basmati or brown rice
1	medium apple, chopped
1 or 2	stalks celery, chopped
1/4 cup	walnuts
4 oz	cooked chicken, chopped
1 tbsp	store-bought light buttermilk dressing, or dressing made with half low-fat yogurt, half low-fat mayonnaise

In bowl, combine rice, apple, celery, walnuts and chicken. Add dressing and toss. Refrigerate until serving.

Makes 1 serving.

Basic Pasta Salad Lunch

1 cup	chopped cooked vegetables (such as broccoli, asparagus, bell peppers, zucchini—whatever's on hand)
1/2 to 1 cup	cooked whole wheat pasta (spirals, shells or similar shape)
1/4 cup	light tomato sauce or any low-fat/non-fat pasta sauce
4 oz	chopped cooked chicken, ground turkey or lean chicken sausage

In bowl, combine vegetables, pasta, sauce and chicken. Refrigerate until serving. Serve either warmed in the microwave or at room temperature.

Makes 1 serving.

Vegetarian Option: Use soy-based ground round instead of the chicken or turkey.

Cottage Cheese and Fruit

1 cup	1% cottage cheese
1 cup	diced fresh fruit, or fruit canned in juice (peaches, apricots or pears)
	Sliced almonds or a few pecans (optional)

In plastic container, combine cottage cheese, fruit and nuts, if using. Seal with tight-fitting lid.

Makes 1 serving.

Fruit Spread Option: Add 1 tbsp double-fruit, no-added-sugar fruit spread instead of the chopped fruit.

The Lunching Out Option

Having lunch out at a restaurant can be tricky. Your friends may tempt you with their orders of fries or pizza. Just walking through the wafting odours of a food court could be enough to make you go off the rails. But you don't want to sit at your desk with a brown bag every day, so here are some tips for keeping your restaurant meal low-G.I.

Eating the G.I. Way in Restaurants

Here are nine tips for keeping your restaurant meal low-G.I.

1. Drink a glass of water before you order or eat. It helps prevent overeating.
2. Ignore the breadbasket. Flatbreads may look thin and diet-ish but, like crackers, they often have hidden trans fats, and they are not low-calorie. Bread and rolls are white flour incarnate. Take a pass.
3. A good addition to your main course is a chunky bean- or vegetable-based soup. But avoid cream-based, noodle or puréed-vegetable soups.
4. When ordering a salad, ask for the dressing on the side; then use only a spoonful of it. Avoid coleslaws, potato salads or anything made with mayonnaise.
5. The only problem with ordering pasta is the size of the portions most restaurants serve. Pasta shouldn't form the base of the meal; it should be a side dish. Most restaurants aren't geared to serving smaller portions, but if you are lunching with a friend, you can order one dish and split it with her. Order whole wheat pasta, if available and make sure the sauce is a low-fat one, such as tomato and basil. No creamy alfredo!
6. If there's a choice between sautéed and grilled, always go for grilled. Sautéeing usually involves oils or butter.

And skip the breaded schnitzels and the tempura shrimp.

7. As it is virtually impossible to get new boiled potatoes, always ask for double vegetables instead. I've requested this substitution hundreds of times and have never been refused.

8. Don't order rice unless it is the long-grain, brown or wild variety. The portion should only cover one quarter of your plate.

9. Eat slowly. Put your fork down between bites. It takes up to half an hour for your stomach to tell your brain when it's had enough. Rushing meals is the most common cause of overeating.

10. Most conventional desserts are red-light; even "diet desserts" will deliver calories. Best to skip it and enjoy a green-light yogurt when you're back at work.

Fast Food

Not so long ago, the idea of getting a green-light lunch at a fast-food outlet was simply laughable. Now, however, partly due to the threat of legal action and a stagnant market share, the major fast-food chains are finally offering some healthy options. Subway has been pioneering the move toward healthy choices for some time, and its initiative has been reflected in its successful growth.

Although things are changing in McDonald's land, fast food is still a minefield. Pizza is red-light all the way thanks to its high-G.I. crust and the saturated fat in the cheese toppings. Hamburgers are also soaked in saturated fat, as are breaded, deep-fried chicken and fish. And all the trimmings—fries, ketchup, shakes and soda—are loaded with fat and sugar. Still, there are a few points of light in this sea of gloom, and I've listed them below. I have put an asterisk beside items that are excessively high in sodium—the fast food industry frequently boosts salt content when they lower the fat in their products to make up for any perceived loss of flavour—which, as we know, can be hazardous to your health. Two asterisks indicates a stratospheric level of salt.

GROUND RULES

1. Always eat burgers open-faced, throwing away the top half of the bun.
2. Always ask for low-fat dressings and use only half of the sachet.

McDonald's

Salads
Chicken Oriental Salad

Dressings
Newman's Own Low Fat Balsamic Dressing*
Mild Chunky Salsa
Newman's Own Low Fat Sesame Thai Dressing*

Burgers and Sandwiches
Whole Wheat Chicken McGrill with BBQ Sauce*

Chicken Protein Platter*
McVeggie Burger*
Turkey BLT
One Chicken Fajita (two is over the line in fat and calories)

Snack
Fruit 'n Yogurt Parfait (hold the granola)

Wendy's

Salads
Mandarin Chicken Salad with Roasted Almonds
Spring Mix Salad with Honey Roasted Pecans

Dressings
Fat Free French Style
Reduced Fat Creamy Ranch
Low Fat Honey Mustard

Burgers
Ultimate Chicken Grill Sandwich* plus side salad

Chili
Large Chili plus side salad

Snack
Junior Frosty (6 oz cup)

Burger King

Salads (hold the Garlic Parmesan Toast on all salads)
Fire-Grilled Chicken or Shrimp Caesar Salad
Fire-Grilled Chicken or Shrimp Garden Salad

Dressings
Ken's Honey Mustard Dressing
Ken's Border Ranch Salad Dressing

Burgers
BK Veggie Burger* plus side salad

Harvey's

Salads
Entree Grilled Chicken Caesar Salad
Entree Grilled Chicken Garden Salad
Entree Caesar Salad

Dressings
Light Caesar
Light Italian

Soups
Beef Barley*
Chicken Noodle*
Harvest Vegetable*

Burgers
Grilled Chicken*
Veggieburger

Swiss Chalet

Meals (hold the flat bread)
Santa Fe Grilled Chicken Salad**
Vegetable Stir Fry on rice*
Chicken Stir Fry on rice**
Quarter Chicken Breast (skinless) Dinner with coleslaw/
    vegetables/corn
Chicken on a Kaiser (white meat)

Dressings
Light Italian Dressing
No-fat Raspberry Vinaigrette

Subway
Note: Best choice of roll is Italian or Wheat.

6-inch Sandwiches with 6 grams of fat or less
Roast Beef*
Oven Roasted Chicken
Turkey Breast*
Turkey Breast & Ham*
Veggie Delite
Sweet Onion Chicken Teriyaki*
Ham*

Deli Style Sandwiches
Ham
Roast Beef
Turkey Breast

Salads
Veggie Delite (side salad)
Grilled Chicken & Baby Spinach

Dressings
Fat-Free Honey Mustard
Fat-Free Wine Vinaigrette
Fat-Free Sweet Onion

Tim Hortons
Ask that your sandwich be made with a whole wheat bun.

Sandwiches
Garden Vegetable
Harvest Turkey Breast
Chicken and Roasted Red Pepper*

Soups
Tim's Own Chicken Noodle*
Vegetable Beef Barley*
Hearty Vegetable*
Turkey and Wild Rice*
Beef Noodle*
Chicken Gumbo*
Tomato Florentine*
Minestrone*

> **Note:** This information was correct at press time. However, as this is a dynamic field, you may wish to check these restaurants' menus or websites from time to time to see if they have expanded their green-light offerings.

Dinner

Dinner, traditionally, is the main meal of the day, and the one where we may have a tendency to overeat. We usually have more time for eating at the end of the day, and we generally feel fatigued as well, which encourages us to consume more. But since we will probably be spending the evening relaxing before going to bed rather than being active, it is important that we don't overdo it. For a complete list of foods, see the Complete G.I. Diet Food Guide on pages 284–94.

PROTEIN			
Meat, Poultry, Fish and Eggs	Breaded fish and seafood	Ground beef (lean)	All fish and seafood (not breaded or canned in oil)
	Fish canned in oil	Lamb (lean cuts)	
	Ground beef (more than 10% fat)	Pork (lean cuts)	Beef (lean cuts)
	Hamburgers	Whole omega-3 eggs	Chicken breast (skinless)
	Hot dogs		Ground beef (extra lean)

	Processed meats Sausages Sushi Whole regular eggs		Lean deli ham Low-cholesterol liquid eggs Turkey breast (skinless) Veal
Dairy	Cheese Cottage cheese (whole or 2%) Milk (whole or 2%) Sour cream Yogurt (whole or 2%)	Cheese (low-fat) Milk (1%) Sour cream (light) Yogurt (low-fat)	Cheese (fat-free) Cottage cheese (1% or fat-free) Fruit yogurt (non-fat with sugar substitute Milk (skim) Soy milk (plain, low-fat)

CARBOHYDRATES

Breads/ Grains	Bagels Baguette/Croissants Cake/Cookies Macaroni & cheese Muffins/Doughnuts Noodles (canned or instant) Pasta filled with cheese or meat Pizza Rice (short-grain, white, instant) Tortillas	Pita (whole wheat) Whole grain breads*	100% stone-ground whole wheat bread* Pasta* (fettuccine, spaghetti, penne, vermicelli, linguine, macaroni) Quinoa Rice (basmati, wild, brown, long-grain) Whole-grain, high-fibre breads (2½–3 g fibre per slice)*

* **Limit serving size (see page 27).**

Fruits/ Vegetables	Broad beans	Apricots	Apples	Lettuce
	French fries	Bananas	Arugula	Mushrooms
	Melons	Beets	Asparagus	Olives*
	Most dried fruit	Corn	Avocado*	Onions
		Kiwi	Beans (green/wax)	Oranges (all varieties)
	Parsnips	Mangoes	Bell peppers	Peaches
	Potatoes (mashed or baked)	Papaya	Blackberries	Pears
		Pineapple	Broccoli	Peas
		Pomegranates	Brussels sprouts	Peppers (hot)
		Potatoes (boiled)	Cabbage	Pickles
		Squash	Carrots	Plums
		Sweet potatoes	Cauliflower	Potatoes (boiled new)
		Yams	Celery	Radishes
			Cherries	Raspberries
			Cucumbers	Snow peas
			Eggplant	Spinach
			Grapefruit	Strawberries
			Grapes	Tomatoes
			Leeks	Zucchini
			Lemons	

FATS

Butter	Corn oil	Almonds*
Hard margarine	Mayonnaise (light)	Canola oil*
Mayonnaise	Most nuts	Hazelnuts
Peanut butter (regular, light)	Salad dressings (light)	Mayonnaise (fat-free)
Salad dressings (regular)	Soft margarine (non-hydrogenated)	Olive oil*
		Pistachios*

* Limit serving size (see page 27).

Tropical oils	Vegetable oils	Salad dressings
Vegetable shortening	Walnuts	(low-fat, low sugar)
		Soft margarine (non-hydrogenated, light)

SOUPS

All cream-based soups	Canned chicken noodle	Chunky bean and vegetable soups
Canned black bean	Canned lentil	(e.g., Campbell's Healthy Request,
Canned green pea	Canned tomato	Healthy Choice, and
Canned puréed vegetable		Too Good To Be True)
Canned split pea		Homemade soups with green-light ingredients

The Protein

No dinner is complete without protein. Whether it is in the form of meat, poultry, seafood, beans or tofu, it should cover no more than one-quarter of your plate. A serving size should be 4 ounces, which is roughly the size of the palm of your hand.

Red Meat

Though most red meat does contain saturated fat, there are a few ways of minimizing it:

- Buy only low-fat meats such as top round beef. For hamburgers or spaghetti sauces, buy extra-lean ground beef. Veal or pork tenderloin are low-fat, too. As for juicy steaks, well, they are juicy because of the fat in them, so they're not a good choice.
- Trim any visible fat from the meat. Even a quarter inch of fat can double the total amount of fat in the meat.
- Broiling or grilling allows the excess fat from the meat to drain off. (Try one of those George Foreman–style fat-draining electric grills.)
- For stovetop cooking, use a non-stick pan with a little vegetable oil spray, rather than oil. The spray goes further.

Poultry
Skinless chicken and turkey breast are excellent green-light choices. In the yellow-light category are skinless thighs, wings and legs, which are higher in fat.

Seafood
Always a good green-light choice. Although certain cold-water fish such as salmon and cod have a relatively high oil content, this oil is omega-3 and is beneficial to your heart health. Shrimp and squid are fine, too, as long as they aren't breaded or battered. Fish and chips, alas, are out.

Beans (legumes)
If you don't think you're into beans, it's time to re-evaluate! Beans are such an excellent source of so many good things: fibre, low-fat protein and "good" carbs that

deliver nutrients while taking their time going through the digestive system. And they are a snap to incorporate into salads and soups to up the protein quotient. Chickpeas, lentils, navy beans, black beans, kidney beans—there's a bean for every day of the week. But watch out for canned pork and beans, which is high in sugar and fat, and avoid canned bean soups, which are processed to the point where their overall G.I. rating is too high.

You will find several delicious recipes using beans in the recipes section of this book.

Tofu

You don't have to be vegetarian to enjoy tofu, which is low in saturated fat and an excellent source of protein. While tofu is not necessarily a thriller on its own, it takes on the flavours of whatever seasonings and sauces it is cooked with. Seasoned tofu scrambles, for instance, are a good substitute for scrambled eggs. Choose soft tofu, which has up to a third less fat than the firm variety.

Textured Vegetable Protein (TVP)

This is not a new device for pre-recording TV shows! TVP is a soy alternative to meat that looks a lot like ground beef, and can be used in the same ways—in lasagna, chili, stir-fries and spaghetti sauce. It's quite tasty and delivers the texture of meat. Our middle son, a vegetarian who has since left the nest, put us onto this adaptable product.

Potatoes, Pasta, Rice

These carbohydrates should cover only one-quarter of the plate. Remember, with potatoes your first choice is boiled small new potatoes. Most other choices, especially baked potatoes or french fries, are red-light. Sweet potatoes are a good lower-G.I. food, but since they tend to come in larger sizes, I suggest you save these for Phase II.

Your serving of pasta should be no more than ¾ cup cooked—just until al dente. If you have rice, make it ⅔ cup cooked basmati, wild, brown or long-grain rice.

Vegetables

Here you can put the measuring cup away. Eat as many vegetables and as much salad as you like; they should be the backbone of your meal. Always include at least two vegetables, and remember to cook them just until tender-crisp. Experiment with something you've never had before. Baby bok choy is delicious grilled, and rapini, a dark green vegetable that looks like broccoli with more leaves, is a nice change. The dark, curly green vegetables such as kale are full of good things, including folic acid.

Greens such as mesclun or baby spinach come conveniently pre-washed in bags. Frozen bags of mixed vegetables are also convenient and inexpensive; you can even toss the veggies into a saucepan, add tomato juice with a dollop of salsa and you have a quick vegetable soup.

Dessert

Yes, dessert is part of the G.I. Diet—at least, the kind that is green-light and good for you. This includes most fruits, and low-fat dairy products, such as yogurt and ice cream sweetened with sugar substitute rather than sugar. All my books have recipes for delicious green-light desserts. Try the Apple Raspberry Coffee Cake or Frozen Ricotta Treat in this one.

Dining Out

Dining out on the G.I. Diet isn't difficult to do since many restaurants have made the switch from butter to olive or vegetable oils and offer more entrees that are broiled or grilled rather than fried, breaded or sauced. They also offer a greater variety of vegetables, salads and fish dishes than they did in the past. All of these changes in the food culture make it easier to dine out the green-light way.

Here are my top ten suggestions for not going astray:

1. Just before you go out, have a small bowl of high-fibre, green-light cold cereal (such as All-Bran) with skim milk and sweetener. I often add a couple of spoonfuls of no-fat/no-sugar fruit yogurt. This will take the edge off your appetite and get some fibre into your digestive system, which will help reduce the G.I. of your upcoming meal.

2.   Once seated in the restaurant, drink a glass of water. It will help you feel fuller. A glass of red wine is a good idea too, but wait till the main course arrives before drinking.

3.   Once the basket of rolls or bread has been passed round the table—which you will ignore—ask the server to remove it. The longer it sits there, the more tempted you will be to dig in.

4.   Order a soup or salad first and tell the server you would like this as soon as possible. This will keep you from sitting there hungry while others are filling up on the bread. For soups, go for vegetable- or bean-based, the chunkier the better. Avoid any that are cream-based, such as vichyssoise. For salads, the golden rule is to keep the dressing on the side. Then you can use a fraction of what the restaurant would normally pour over the greens. And please avoid Caesar salads, which come pre-dressed and often pack as many calories as a burger.

5.   Since you probably won't get boiled new potatoes and can't be sure of what type of rice is being served, ask for double vegetables instead. I have yet to find a restaurant that won't oblige.

6.   Stick with low-fat cuts of meat or poultry. If necessary, you can remove the skin. Duck is usually too high in fat. Fish and shellfish are excellent choices but shouldn't be breaded or battered. Tempura is more fat and flour than filling. And remember that servings tend to be generous

in restaurants, so eat only 4 to 6 ounces (a pack of cards) and leave the rest.

7. As with salads, ask for any sauces to be put on the side.

8. For dessert, fresh fruit and berries, if available, are your best choice—without the ice cream. Most other choices are a dietary disaster. My advice is to avoid dessert. If a birthday cake is being passed around, share your piece with someone. A couple of forkfuls or so along with your coffee should get you off the hook, with minimal dietary damage!

9. Only order decaffeinated coffee. Skim-milk decaf cappuccino is our family's favourite choice.

10. Finally, and perhaps most important, eat slowly. In the eighteenth century, Dr. Samuel Johnson famously advised chewing one's food thirty-two times before swallowing! That's going a little overboard, but at least put your fork down between mouthfuls. The stomach can take up to half an hour to let the brain know it feels full. So if you eat quickly, you may be shovelling in more food than you require, till the brain finally says stop. You will also be able to savour your meal longer.

Snacks

Keep your digestive system busy and your energy up with three between-meal snacks a day—one mid-morning, one mid-afternoon and one before bed.

SNACKS		
Bagels	Bananas	Almonds**
Candy	Dark chocolate (70% cocoa)	Applesauce (unsweetened)
Cookies		
Crackers	Ice cream (low-fat)	Canned peaches/pears in juice or water
Doughnuts	Most nuts	
Flavoured gelatin (all varieties)	Popcorn (air popped)	Cottage cheese (1% or fat-free)
French fries		Extra low-fat cheese (e.g., Laughing Cow Light, Boursin Light)
Ice cream		
Muffins (commercial)		Fruit yogurt (non-fat with sugar substitute)
Popcorn (regular)		
Potato chips		Food bars*
Pretzels		Hazelnuts**
Pudding		Homemade green-light snacks (see pp. 268–78)
Raisins		
Rice cakes		
Sorbet		Ice cream (low-fat and no added sugar, e.g., Breyers Premium Fat-Free, Nestlé Legend)
Tortilla chips		
Trail mix		
White bread		Most fresh fruit
		Most fresh vegetables
		Pickles
		Pumpkin seeds
		Sugar-free hard candies
		Sunflower seeds

* 180–225 calorie bars, e.g., Zone or Balance Bars; ½ bar per serving.
** Limit serving size (see page 27).

Try to eat balanced snacks that include a bit of protein and carbohydrates. For example, a piece of fruit with a few nuts, or cottage cheese with celery sticks.

A convenient snack for when you're on the go is half an energy bar. Be careful when choosing one: most of them are full of cereal and sugar. The ones to look for list 20 to 30 grams of carbohydrates, 12 to 15 grams of protein and 5 grams of fat. Balance and ZonePerfect bars are two examples.

Keep in mind that many snacks and desserts labelled "low-fat" or "sugar-free" aren't necessarily green-light. Sugar-free instant puddings or "low-fat" muffins are still high-G.I. because they contain highly processed grains.

Dear Rick,

Really, this email is just a gloat! I have never managed to stick to a diet longer than three or four weeks, and have always felt terribly hard done by on them. However, I have now been on the G.I. Diet for eight weeks, and I feel great. I started at 160 pounds and am now at 142, and if I do say so myself, I look the best I have since I was an awful lot younger! This diet has not only changed my eating habits, but has improved my self-confidence greatly. Eating the G.I. way is so easy, and in fact I struggle to eat three meals and three snacks a day, as I feel so satisfied with the portions I do eat. I've managed to convert my mother and best friend to the G.I. way, not by lecturing them, but just by shrinking every time I see them without any perceived effort!

Heather

Beverages

Because liquids don't trip our satiety mechanisms, it's a waste to take in calories through them. And many beverages are high-calorie. Juice, for example, is a processed product, and has a much higher G.I. than the fruit or vegetable it is made from. A glass of orange juice contains nearly two and a half times the calories of a fresh orange! So eat the fruit or vegetable rather than drink its juice. That way you'll get all the benefits of its nutrients and fibre while consuming fewer calories.

As well, we should stay away from any beverage that contains added sugar or caffeine. As I explained earlier, caffeine stimulates insulin, which leads to us feeling hungry. So, no coffee or soft drinks containing caffeine in Phase I.

That said, fluids are an important part of any diet—I'm sure you're all familiar with the eight-glasses-a-day prescription. The following are your best green-light choices:

Water

The cheapest, easiest and best thing to drink is plain water. Seventy percent of our body consists of water, which is needed for digestion, circulation, regulation of body temperature, lubrication of joints and healthy skin. We can live for months without food, but we can only survive a few days without water.

Don't feel you have to drink eight glasses of water a day in addition to other beverages. Milk, tea and soft drinks all

contribute to the eight-glass-a-day recommendation. But
do try to drink a glass of water before each meal—it will
help you feel fuller so that you don't overeat.

Skim milk

After a skeptical start, I've grown to really enjoy skim milk,
and I like to drink it with breakfast and lunch, which tend
to be a little short on protein. Skim milk is an ideal green-
light food.

Soft Drinks

If you're used to drinking soft drinks, you can still enjoy
the sugar- and caffeine-free diet ones. People often treat
regular soft drinks and fruit juices as non-foods, but this
is how extra calories slip by us.

Tea

Although black and green teas do contain caffeine, the
amount is only about a third of that of coffee. And tea has
health benefits as well. Black and green teas contain
antioxidant properties that help prevent heart disease and
Alzheimer's. In fact, tea has more flavonoids (antioxidants) than any vegetable tested. Two cups of black or
green tea have the same amount of antioxidants as 7 cups
of orange juice or 28 cups of apple juice.

So tea in moderation is fine—minus the sugar and
cream, of course. Try some new varieties: Darjeeling, Earl
Grey, English Breakfast or spicy chai (with sugar substitute). Herbal teas are also a green-light option, though

they lack the flavonoids. Iced tea is also acceptable if it's sugar-free.

Alcohol

Alcohol is generally a disaster for any weight-loss program. It puts your blood sugar on a roller coaster: you go up and feel great, then come down and feel like having another drink, or eating the whole bowl of peanuts. Alcohol also contains a lot of calories.

On the other hand, a little red wine can be beneficial for your heart health, and in Phase II, we encourage you to have a glass of wine with dinner. In Phase I, however, put away the corkscrew and the ice cube tray.

TO SUM UP

- In Phase I, eat only green-light foods—three meals and three balanced snacks per day.
- Drink plenty of fluids, including an eight-ounce glass of water with meals and snacks (but no caffeine or alcohol).
- Pay attention to portion size: palm of your hand for protein, and a quarter plate for pasta, potatoes or rice. Use common sense and eat moderate amounts.
- Don't get discouraged by lapses. If you eat green-light 90 percent of the time, you'll still be fine.

CHAPTER FIVE

Frequently Asked Questions

Q. How is the G.I. Diet different from the Atkins Diet? Can I switch from Atkins to the G.I. Diet without gaining weight?

A. The difference is like night and day. The Atkins diet is based on high protein, including animal fat (saturated fat) and very low consumption of carbohydrates. The idea is that when the body is deprived of carbohydrates as the primary source of energy, it will be forced to break down fat instead. The process is called ketosis, and over time, it can cause serious long-term health issues, such as osteoporosis and kidney damage. The high saturated fat content of the Atkins diet is also associated with a higher risk of heart disease, stroke, Alzheimer's and colon and prostate cancers.

Yes, you will probably lose weight on the Atkins diet. But many people gain it all back again, and this yo-yo effect tends to make it even harder to lose weight and keep it off the next time you embark on a diet.

The G.I. Diet is just the reverse. Carbohydrates such as fruit, vegetables, whole grains, beans and low-fat dairy products are all encouraged, not limited, while saturated fat is virtually eliminated. If there is one thing that all the health, medical and nutritional authorities agree upon, it is that a diet rich in vegetables, fruits, nuts, legumes, lean meat/fish and whole grains is essential for long-term good health. And that's the G.I. Diet in a nutshell.

As high-protein diets are diuretic, you will likely gain some temporary weight when you switch to the G.I. Diet and your body rehydrates. When things settle down after a couple of weeks, you will resume your weight loss, while giving your body the nutrition it needs for long-term health.

Q. Is this a good diet for people with diabetes?

A. The key to controlling diabetes is to control blood sugar levels. It is the instability of blood sugar levels and the diabetic's inability to produce enough insulin to remove the sugar from the bloodstream that creates the medical condition called hyperglycemia. If left uncontrolled, this can lead to death. The glycemic index was originally developed by Dr. David Jenkins to address the issue of which carbohydrates diabetics could eat to minimize hyperglycemia (high blood sugar levels). This is why diabetics find the G.I. Diet so effective in the management of their disease. Many have been able to reduce their medications and, in some cases, even eliminate them. As being overweight is one of the key reasons people develop diabetes in the first place, losing weight with the G.I. Diet provides a further added benefit. The Canadian Diabetes Association, in its house magazine, *Dialogue,* recommended the G.I. Diet as the best choice for diabetics among the leading popular diets.

Q. Will the G.I. Diet work for vegetarians?

A. The G.I. Diet is an excellent way for vegetarians to eat. Simply replace meat, chicken and fish with alternate protein sources: beans, nuts and soy products such as tofu or tempeh. The G.I. Diet's emphasis on fruits, vegetables, legumes, nuts and low-fat dairy ensures that most nutritional needs are met in spades. A multivitamin is advisable to ensure sufficient B vitamins, which are principally found in meats. (For more on vegetarians' and vegans' nutritional needs, see pages 162–64.)

Q. I seem to have hit a plateau. What should I do?

A. This is a common complaint. The thing to remember is that you never lose weight on a steady and unvarying basis. You may drop twenty pounds and then reach a point when your weight doesn't budge for a week or even two or three.

As we mentioned earlier, the average weight loss target is one pound per week, depending on what percent of body weight you want to lose. So count the number of weeks you have been eating the low-G.I. way and divide them into the number of pounds lost. This will give you your average weekly weight loss, which you will find almost invariably hits your objective of one pound per week. This means you're on target and your weight loss will kick in again soon.

If you are falling behind on your average or the plateau lasts more than a couple of weeks, then you need to check the serving sizes of your green-light foods, particularly the ones we've specified serving sizes for, such as potatoes, pasta, rice and nuts (see page 27). Check that you are following the guidelines.

With all other low-G.I. products, make sure moderation is your motto. Consuming a 500-gram tub of low-fat yogurt at a sitting or eating twelve apples a day is clearly not moderation. Be honest with yourself and review what you are currently eating. Keep a food diary for a few days. The only person you are kidding is yourself!

Q. How is the G.I. Diet different from the South Beach Diet?

A. Broadly speaking, there are many similarities between the approach taken in the South Beach Diet and the G.I. Diet. But there are a couple of significant differences. First, the South Beach Diet has one extra stage; its Phase I is a kind of crash diet. The G.I. Diet does not require or recommend a crash diet. Second, the G.I. Diet is simpler and easier to use than the South Beach Diet. All the calculations have been done for you. Simply follow the colour-coded charts.

Q. Is it true that the G.I. Diet can help relieve depression?

A. While the G.I. Diet cannot claim to relieve clinical depression, it can alleviate one of the key compounding factors: blood sugar levels.

Q. What if I fall off the wagon?

A. This is a primary concern of readers, but it doesn't need to be. If you can be on the program for 90 percent of the time, that's just fine. The worst that can happen is that you will delay reaching your weight target by a week or two. This is a real-world way of eating that recognizes the realities of hectic schedules and social pressures, of eating on the run and of the sheer temptation to binge on occasion. Luckily, the G.I. plan has a built-in warning signal whenever you go off the rails. After a few weeks of eating the low-G.I. way and keeping your blood sugar levels steady, your body will react with alarm to any sudden onslaught of high-G.I. foods. You will end up feeling bloated, tired and irritable. Believe me, it will be a relief to climb back on board the green-light wagon.

Q. Aren't aspartame and other sugar substitutes bad for your health?

A. A great deal of misinformation has been spread about sugar substitutes—driven mainly by the sugar lobby in the United States. All the major government and health agencies worldwide have approved the use of sweeteners and sugar substitutes, and not a single peer-reviewed (scholarly) study has identified any health risks. For those who are still concerned about the safety of artificial sweeteners, there is a comprehensive rundown on sugar substitutes in the U.S. Food and Drug Administration's newsletter, called *FDA Consumer* (see www.fda.gov). If you're sensitive to aspartame, check out such alternatives as sucralose (Splenda), which is our personal favourite.

Q. Why aren't certain low-calorie foods such as rice cakes or sugar-free Jell-O green-light?

A. Although they don't have a lot of calories, they are digested quickly, leaving you looking for more food to keep your digestive system busy. The whole idea behind the G.I. Diet is to eat low-G.I. foods that keep you feeling full for longer, i.e., that are more satiating. Try to stick to green-light snacks, which are far more nutritious and satisfying.

Q. Is the G.I. Diet suitable for people who do extended workouts?

A. Absolutely. Other than ensuring your serving sizes are delivering sufficient calories to meet your higher calorie needs, the only modification is the need to replenish your glycogen levels (the body's short-term glucose storage for muscles), which can get depleted during a prolonged workout. Following your workout with a sugar-based drink such as Gatorade is ideal. Otherwise you may feel lethargic.

Q. I have to travel a lot for business—how can I stay on track with the G.I. Diet?

A. Follow the green-light guidelines for eating out on pages 69–76 and 83–85. On planes, vegetarian meals are often fresher and more green-light than the standard entrees, which tend to be served with sauces. Call ahead to book them, or bring along your own supply of almonds, a nutrition bar, a small tub of yogurt or some fruit so that you won't be tempted by the pretzels and cookies handed out mid-flight.

Airports are nutritional deserts, but usually you can scout the cafeterias for a bit of fruit. Some airports now have juice and smoothie concessions, and in the southern states, you can always find a bean burrito to tide you over. Basically, try to schedule your meals so you never find yourself hungry in an airport. You'll save money this way, too.

CHAPTER SIX

Phase II

Well, you've made it. Congratulations! You've hit your target weight, you're digging out clothes you thought you'd never get into again, and you're finally on good terms with your full-length mirror. I hope you are relishing the new you and making the most of your increased energy. Now that you've graduated from Phase I, you can ease up a bit on limiting portion and serving sizes and start adding some yellow-light foods to your diet. The idea here is to get comfortable with your G.I. program; this is how you're going to eat for the rest of your life.

Of course, Phase II is also the danger zone, the stage when most diets go off the rails. Most people think that when they reach their weight-loss goal, they can just drop the diet and go back to their old eating habits. And frankly, when I take a close look at what many of these diets expect you to live on, I can understand why people can't stick to them for long.

The reality is that with some modifications, the G.I. program is your diet for life. But this shouldn't be a hardship, because the G.I. Diet was designed to give you a huge range of healthy choices, so you won't feel hungry, bored or unsatisfied. By now, you will know how to navigate your green-light way around the supermarket aisles, you will know how to decipher food labels, and cooking the green-light way will be second nature. But the strangest thing may be that you are not even tempted to revert to your old ways. If you should fall prey to a double cheeseburger, you will be dismayed at how heavy, sluggish and ungratified you feel afterward. You will be too attached to your new feeling of lightness and level of energy to abandon them.

Before we look at some of the new options open to you in Phase II, a word of caution: your body can now function on less food than it did before you started. Why? Because you're lighter now, and so your body requires

Dear Rick,
I purposely waited a year before writing to you because I wanted to be sure that this was really a sustainable change in eating patterns. I can now confirm that the G.I. Diet is totally sustainable; in fact, I feel more satisfied and less hungry than ever. I cannot conceive of going back to my old way of eating and do not have the slightest desire to do so. My wife feels the same way. My blood pressure is lower, I no longer have any heartburn, and my workouts are fantastic and fun.
Thanks,
Michael

fewer calories. Also, your metabolism has become more efficient, and your body has learned to do more with fewer calories than in its old spendthrift days. Keeping these two developments in mind, add a few more calories in Phase II, but don't go berserk. Don't make any significant changes in your serving sizes, and remember to make yellow-light foods the exception rather than the rule. This way you will keep the balance between the calories you're consuming and the calories you're expending—and that is the secret to maintaining your new weight.

As you modestly increase portions of foods that you particularly enjoy and include some yellow-light items as a treat, keep monitoring your weight weekly, and adjust your servings up or down until your weight stays stable. This may take a few weeks of experimentation, but when you've reached the magic balance and can stay there comfortably, that's the formula for the rest of your days (give or take a piece of wedding cake or a birthday indulgence).

Here are some ideas of how you might alter the way you eat in Phase II.

Breakfast
- Increase cereal serving size from half a cup to two-thirds of a cup.
- Add a slice of 100% whole grain toast and a pat of margarine.
- Double the amount of sliced almonds on your cereal.
- Enjoy an extra slice of back bacon.
- Have a glass of unsweetened juice now and then.

- Add one of the yellow-light fruits—a banana or apricot—
to your cereal.
- Go caffeinated in the coffee department, if you like, but try
to keep it to one cup a day.

Lunch

I suggest you continue to eat lunch as you did in Phase I,
as this is the one meal that already contained some com-
promises in the weight-loss portion of the program.

Dinner

- Add another boiled new potato.
- Increase the pasta serving from ¾ cup to 1 cup.
- As a special treat, have a 6-ounce steak instead of a
4-ounce one.
- Eat a few more olives and nuts—but only a few!
- Try a cob of sweet corn with a dab of margarine.
- Add a slice of high-fibre bread or crispbread.
- Enjoy a yellow-light cut of lamb or pork.

Snacks

- Have a maximum of 2 cups of air-popped popcorn.
- Increase your serving size of nuts to 10 or 12.
- Enjoy a square or two of 70 percent dark chocolate (see
below).
- Have a banana.
- Indulge in a scoop of low-fat ice cream or frozen yogurt.

Chocolate

For many of us, living without chocolate is not living. The
good news is that in Phase II, some chocolate—the right

sort of chocolate in the right amount—is acceptable. You may have heard that chocolate, like red wine, contains natural elements that help keep the arteries clear—but that's probably not your main motive for eating it. Chocolate combines fat, sugar and cocoa, all three of which please the palate. But most chocolate contains too much saturated fat and sugar, which keeps it deep in the red-light zone. Chocolate with a high cocoa content (70 percent or more) delivers more chocolate intensity per ounce, which means that even a square or two is satisfying. A square or two can give chocoholics the fix they need.

Alcohol

The other good news in Phase II is that a glass of red wine is allowed with dinner. Medical research indicates that red wine, which is rich in flavonoids, can help reduce your risk of heart disease and stroke. Just because one glass is beneficial, however, doesn't mean that two or three is even better for you. Immoderate drinking undoes any health benefits, and alcohol is always calorific. One glass of wine (5 ounces maximum) provides the optimum benefit.

Apart from red wine, keep your consumption of alcohol to a minimum. I realize that this can be difficult, since drinking is so often a part of social occasions and celebrations. An occasional lapse won't do a lot of harm, but it's easy to get carried away. There are various strategies for getting around the social pressure to drink: you can graciously accept that glass of wine or cocktail, raise it in a toast, take a sip, and then discreetly leave it on the nearest buffet table. Faced with a tray of vodka martinis and glasses of red wine, stick with the wine, which lasts longer. My wife, Ruth, drinks spritzers (wine mixed with soda water) on special occasions. And if you add lots of ice to your spritzer, you can reduce the alcohol even further while still joining in the party spirit. Whatever strategy you choose, always try to eat some food with your drink, even if it has to be a forbidden piece of cheese. The fat will slow down the absorption of the alcohol and minimize its impact. (Of course, better to gravitate to the vegetable tray, but an emergency canapé won't be the ruin of you.)

Motivation

The way you now look, the response of your family and friends, and the way you feel will all help motivate you to keep to the green-light path. Going back to your old eating habits will seem less like a temptation than a way to undermine all the good things that weight loss has brought you so far. But if you should ever need reinforcement, or if your resolve begins to waver, here are a couple of "cures" you can try:

The $10 Cure

This is the food version of what immigrants (like me) used to call the "$1,000 Cure." Whenever a new arrival, after a long cold winter in Canada, started to pine for "the old country," the cure was to get on a plane and go home for a week. All the reasons that originally persuaded the person to emigrate would come crashing back, until the thought of flying back to Canada began to look pretty good again.

With food, the cure costs less—say, $10. When you pine for "the old food," try this: go out for lunch with some friends and order a high-G.I. meal—a slice of double-cheese pizza, a Coke and a brownie. Your mouth may enjoy it, but I guarantee that a couple hours later you'll be desperate for a nap, feeling lethargic and lousy. And that's not even factoring in your guilt. Trust me, you won't want to repeat the experience!

The Shopping Bag Cure

For this motivator, fill up a plastic shopping bag—or two if necessary —with some books or cans of food. Step on the scales and keep adding books or cans until you reach your original weight. Then simply walk up and down the stairs a few times. You'll be so glad that this weight is something you can put down. No wonder you used to be so low on energy and your back and joints ached.

One reader in England wrote to say that when she lost 70 pounds, she tried the Shopping Bag Cure. She had to fill four bags, and they were so heavy she couldn't even pick them up—and that was what she had been carrying around all the time!

Of course, Phase II is not, and shouldn't be, a straitjacket. If you live 90 percent within the guidelines of the diet, you are doing well. The idea that certain foods are completely and forever forbidden would drive you, sooner or later, back into their clutches. With the G.I. Diet, you are in control of what you eat, and that includes (with discipline, moderation and common sense) almost everything.

TO SUM UP
- In Phase II, use moderation and common sense in adjusting portions and servings.
- Don't view Phase II as a straitjacket. Occasional lapses are fine.
- For motivation, try the $10 Cure or the Shopping Bag Cure.

PART II

The Family

CHAPTER SEVEN

The Special
Nutritional
Needs of Women

I have asked my wife, Ruth, to author this chapter to provide a woman's perspective and to share her knowledge. Ruth is professor emeritus at the University of Toronto with a special interest in women's health.

Most of the readers who email Rick about their experiences with the G.I. Diet are women. This is hardly surprising, given the relationship between popular culture, women's body image, weight and food. In the 1994–95 National Population Health Survey conducted by Statistics Canada, 40 percent of women reported they were trying to lose weight compared to 24 percent of men. Of those survey respondents who were overweight, 70 percent of women reported they were trying to lose weight, while only 48 percent of men did. Aside from all the sociological reasons why women are more concerned about their weight than men, the issue of eating is always going to be more complicated for women because of our physiology, the fact that we can bear children. The beginning of our reproductive life, the onset of menstruation, and the end, menopause, bring hormonal changes and resultant nutritional and weight control concerns. And of course, many women never experience any weight problems until after pregnancy. Let's look at these specific dietary issues in turn.

Women's Metabolism

We've had a number of emails from women who tell us about their frustration when their husbands join them on the G.I. Diet. They report that the men lose weight faster than they do. Yes, this can happen—and it can be discouraging!

It's not that men are stricter or more disciplined. The reality is that men and women have different metabolisms, and this affects the rate at which our bodies turn food into fuel. Women also have more body fat than men; that's what accounts for our curves. In general, women have about 27 percent body fat, compared with an average of 15 percent in men. Men also have more muscle tissue than women, and muscle burns more calories than fat. (That's why your husband can fall off the diet now and then and not pay the price, whereas one piece of birthday cake seems to show up the next morning on your scales.)

Why do women have this extra padding of fat? It plays a role in the natural processes of ovulation, menstruation and reproduction. Fat helps the production and circulation of estrogen, and ensures that a pregnant woman has some reserves of energy to nourish new life. A woman's body is always, on some level, operating with the potential to sustain another life, even if conception or reproduction never occurs. But what works so beautifully for child-bearing may be counterproductive for trying to lose weight.

Hormones play a huge role in weight control and cravings at different stages of your life. They can affect what you want to eat during pregnancy, and when the levels shift once again during menopause, hormones can affect blood sugar levels and play havoc with weight control. Then there is the issue of appetite changes affected by PMS (see below). This goes along with a temporary spike in weight (and feeling bloated) that some women experience premenstrually. There are days when women not only "feel fat," but their weight truly does fluctuate, even when their eating habits don't.

Aging affects metabolism as well. Women, on average, gain ten pounds per decade, unless they adjust their eating accordingly. The older you get, the fewer calories your body requires. If you're sixty-eight and can't seem to stop gaining weight, take a look at your portions; you shouldn't be eating the same amount you were eating at the age of fifty. (For more on the senior years, turn to chapter ten.)

How Diet Affects Menstruation

The age at which girls begin to menstruate has gradually been coming down. Now girls sometimes get their period at the age of nine or ten. But although the menarche officially marks the time when the female body is ready for reproduction, it's important to remember that at this age a girl is still growing, and her body isn't "finished" yet. Young girls continue to need the right nutrition to feed both body and brain. Those who become diet-crazy and severely restrict their eating can put their overall development at risk and stress major organs such as the heart and kidneys (see more on eating disorders on pages 158–60).

It's important for girls and women to have enough fat (preferably the good kind) in their diet; otherwise menstruation will be interrupted. For women with a BMI of less than 18, periods are likely to cease, and this could indicate that other aspects of health are at risk, too. For instance, during the menstrual years, women need to make sure they get enough iron, about 15 milligrams a day, to replace what they lose during their periods. Women need one and a half times as much iron as men do each day. Iron is an essential element of hemoglobin, which helps carry oxygen in our blood. When iron levels are too low, we can develop anemia, which brings fatigue, irritability and pallor.

Women who are pregnant or breast-feeding are particularly at risk for low iron. Approximately 10 percent of women in North America are iron-deficient, and this number rises to 25 percent during pregnancy. A recent study from the University of Pennsylvania suggests that even mild iron depletion can affect our concentration and ability to think. After improving their iron levels, women with minor deficiencies raised their scores on tests that evaluated attention, short-term and long-term memory.

Normally, if our diet is a good one, we can get all the iron we need from the foods we eat. Red meats (lean cuts of beef or extra-lean ground beef), eggs and dark green leafy vegetables such as broccoli and spinach are excellent sources. Seafood and legumes also contain some iron.

Menstruation can affect appetite, cravings and blood sugar levels. Such symptoms as a desire for sugar, irritability and mood swings may show up in the second half of the menstrual cycle, when estrogen levels drop and progesterone rises. (In the first half, estrogen dominates and progesterone levels are lower.) Early research into the biochemistry of PMS—which wasn't recognized as a physiological reality until recently—discovered that diet can make a difference in the severity of PMS. Dr. Katharine Dalton, a pioneering British researcher in this area, found that a diet that emphasizes complex carbohydrates and low-fat foods can diminish problems associated with PMS. She also recommends eating three meals and three snacks a day. In other words, the anti-PMS diet perfectly matches the G.I. Diet. High-G.I. foods are digested quickly, spiking glucose levels which then quickly plummet, exacerbating symptoms such as depression, irritability and mood swings. Keeping sugar levels stable is critical to managing mood, headaches and food cravings.

Recent research has also shown that a diet rich in calcium (1,200 milligrams a day) can help prevent or relieve the severity of PMS. Make sure that skim milk and low-fat yogurt are part of your G.I. Diet.

Food, Dieting and Pregnancy

We all know that pregnancy is a time when we should pay special attention to our diet and nutrition. But don't forget that diet can also affect fertility, and that proper nutrition for your child begins at conception. Don't postpone; start eating healthily as soon as you start thinking about getting pregnant.

Since being overweight increases the risk of health problems and complications during pregnancy, if your BMI is 25 or over, you would be well advised to try to lose some weight before you get pregnant. At the same time, however, adequate body fat is essential for conception, so a too-low BMI is not ideal either. Too much strenuous exercise can lower body fat to the point where it interferes with your ability to conceive. Don't take this as an excuse to turn into a couch potato, but perhaps delay training for a marathon.

If you're hoping to get pregnant, refrain from smoking and drinking alcohol, which can have devastating effects on a baby, lowering birth weight and possibly causing fetal alcohol syndrome. Research also tells us that women trying to conceive should be sure to get enough folic acid, 400 micrograms (0.4 milligrams) daily. Folic acid is critical for healthy neural tube development (an early part of normal brain growth), which often occurs in the fetus before a woman even knows she's pregnant.

It goes without saying that you are *supposed* to gain weight during pregnancy—most women gain twenty-two to thirty pounds. But if you are overweight when you become pregnant, you can safely follow Phase I of the G.I. Diet. All the foods normally recommended during pregnancy, such as fresh fruit and vegetables, whole grains, lean meat, fish and low-fat dairy products, are staples of Phase I. However, if this way of eating is a radical shift for you, you should talk to your doctor before embarking on the program.

If your BMI is in the healthy range, Phase II of the G.I. Diet is a healthy way for you to eat during pregnancy. It will provide you and your child with the necessary calories and nutrition and help you avoid gaining too much weight. But there are some additional dietary considerations during this special time:

Fish
Fish is an excellent source of protein and omega-3 fats, and evidence suggests that it reduces the risk of premature birth, so be sure to include it in your diet. Unfortunately, some fish—the larger species—have been

found to contain high levels of mercury, which can damage your baby's brain. Avoid shark, swordfish, king mackerel, tilefish and fresh and frozen tuna when trying to get pregnant and during the first trimester, and limit these to no more than one serving a month thereafter. Canned albacore tuna appears to be safe in amounts not exceeding 6 ounces a week. And you can safely consume up to 12 ounces a week of fish such as fresh, frozen and canned salmon, halibut, sardines, mackerel and trout, and seafood such as shrimp, squid and octopus. Just make sure that the fish and seafood you eat are fully cooked to kill any disease-causing bacteria or parasites. This is not the time for that barely seared tuna or raw oysters. Also avoid smoked fish unless it has been cooked in a dish like a casserole.

Aspartame
Though the sugar substitute aspartame has been approved for use by government regulators, no safety limits have yet been established for pregnant or nursing women. Our advice then is to use it sparingly. We prefer Splenda (sucralose), which is actually derived from sugar, and can be found in some brands of diet soft drinks, non-fat ice cream and non-fat, sugar-free yogurt—just check labels. Alternatively, you can buy low- or non-fat plain, unsweetened yogurt and sweeten it yourself with fresh fruit or extra-fruit jam.

Listeriosis

Listeriosis is a form of food poisoning that is especially dangerous during pregnancy, possibly leading to premature delivery or miscarriage. It can be caused by unpasteurized cheeses and other dairy products, packaged luncheon meats and deli meats, and raw and undercooked eggs. So avoid eating unpasteurized dairy products, including soft cheeses such as brie, camembert, Roquefort, feta and goat cheese—which are only used sparingly as a flavour inhancer on the G.I. Diet anyway. If you are eating out, ask whether any unpasteurized cheese has been added to the dishes. Don't eat raw or undercooked eggs and avoid luncheon meats unless they have been heated until hot.

Caffeine

Although research indicates that moderate amounts of caffeine (less than 300 milligrams a day from all sources, including coffee, tea, soft drinks and chocolate) won't harm your baby, caffeine does cross the placenta and some studies have linked it to attention deficit disorder and migraines. Some women find they naturally go off coffee and tea very early in pregnancy, although this aversion can mysteriously wear off by the late stages, when the appetite for old habits may return. If you absolutely must, limit yourself to one cup a day, or have black or green tea, which have beneficial antioxidants and less caffeine than coffee. If you like herbal tea, be cautious: some herbs are not compatible with pregnancy or nursing. Check labels.

Alcohol

Although Phase II of the G.I. Diet allows you to enjoy a glass of red wine with dinner, no safe level of alcohol consumption has been established for pregnancy. It is best, then, to avoid it.

Dear Rick,

When I bought the G.I. Diet, my story was no different than that of millions of others. I had always battled with my weight, but was never truly overweight until I hit my thirties. The G.I. Diet was the easiest and best weight management program I've ever tried. I lost 20 pounds in four months, and I continue to rave about it to anyone who will listen. Every time I read the G.I. newsletter, I'm glad to hear of other people's success stories. It never occurred to me that mine was remotely special in comparison with theirs—until now. I'm five months pregnant with my first child, and the changes that the G.I. Diet made to my eating habits have made a remarkable difference. I was always terrified that I would be one of those women who gained more than just "baby weight." Instead, my Phase II eating habits have helped me keep my weight gain in the proper range. I also have not had any trouble with gestational diabetes and I have tons of energy! So, Rick, thank you from me, and thank you from my little one on the way!

Dawn

"Eating for Two"

Don't let the notion that you are "eating for two" become your excuse to double your calories. Your baby will not "use up" your extra body fat. Eating three low-G.I. meals and three snacks a day will keep your glucose levels and energy stable and help to control your appetite. But what happens if you start experiencing cravings? Some women crave sweet (chocolate) while others crave sour (the classic one being pickles). I remember craving strawberries. It's not clear why this happens, but it may have something to do with our bodies trying to fulfill a need for a particular nutrient. Try to identify the flavour you are craving and find a green-light food that will assuage it. For example, if you want something sweet and creamy, try low-fat ice cream with no added sugar; if you want something sour, have a dill pickle or a salad with lemon juice sprinkled over it. If it's peanut butter you're desperately hankering for, go ahead and savour one tablespoon a day of the natural kind, which contains only peanuts. If it's chocolate that you want, let one square dissolve in your mouth. Be careful not to overdo it.

Common Conditions and Diet During Pregnancy

Morning Sickness

Morning sickness can be a problem for some women during the first trimester. Often particular foods or strong smells trigger nausea; it might be frying bacon or the smell of chicken noodle soup. You'll know when you experience it! Try to find an eating pattern that works for you. Sometimes it helps to eat a piece of whole wheat toast or a cracker before you get up. Or you may find it easier to start the day with a snack, then have breakfast later. If eating full meals puts you off, you might need to forget about meals and slowly graze all day (but keep track, so you know your total daily intake). Drink fluids slowly or drink between meals. Keep a bottle of water handy throughout the day so you can take small sips and stay hydrated, even when the thought of eating turns your stomach. Water will also keep your kidneys functioning well, minimize constipation and make you feel better.

Morning sickness usually abates by week eleven or twelve. For some unlucky women, however, it can persist throughout the pregnancy. If you are vomiting a lot, you should talk to your doctor, since you may be losing essential nutrients (not to mention feeling awful).

Hemorrhoids
Hemorrhoids are another condition that pregnancy can aggravate. The best way to prevent them is to avoid becoming constipated; eat lots of fibre, vegetables and fresh fruit; and drink plenty of water.

Heartburn
Heartburn can develop during the last trimester, and is usually experienced at night. The baby is growing, and your uterus is now pressing against your stomach,

demanding space. But there are many tricks to minimize or eliminate heartburn, beginning with avoiding spicy and acidic foods. Tomato sauce, citrus fruits, curries, chocolate and decaf coffee can all trigger heartburn. So can eating too quickly or feeling stressed.

The key to preventing heartburn at night is to eat an early light dinner and to snack lightly (if at all) after 8 P.M. Unlike during the first trimester, when you may have opted for light breakfasts, this might be the time to front-load your day with a larger breakfast, followed by a normal lunch and a light dinner. Believe it or not, raising the head of your bed an inch or two on blocks, or adding an extra pillow to keep the top of your body elevated, can help as well. It's better to treat heartburn through watching when, what and how much you eat rather than relying on antacids or prescription acid inhibitors.

Weight Loss After Pregnancy

Congratulations, you have a new baby, and a new adventure has begun! Though you will lose weight after giving birth—on average between 10 and 20 pounds in the first couple of weeks—many women are dismayed to find that they don't immediately return to their pre-pregnancy weight. Be patient; your body has just undergone nine months of tremendous changes and will need time, as many as nine months, to recover. Your main concern right now should be looking after your health, making sure to eat right and get all the nutrients you, and your baby if you are breast-feeding, need. If you were on Phase II of the

G.I. Diet during pregnancy and are breast-feeding, you can continue with it now (see more on this below). If you have decided not to breast-feed, you can start with Phase I. If, however, the G.I. Diet represents a major change in your eating habits, let your body recover from the birth for three to four weeks before embarking on it. You can also gradually introduce moderate exercise once your body is up to it.

Breast-Feeding

Breast-feeding contributes a great deal to the health of your baby, and most experts recommend you do so for about six months. Research suggests that the longer you breast-feed, the less chances your child will have of developing food allergies, and breast milk seems to offer additional immune-strengthening benefits as well. It is worth noting that women who breast-feed use up the extra body fat gained during pregnancy faster than women who don't.

Many women who are breast-feeding ask whether they can remain on the G.I. Diet while they nurse their babies—and yes, they can safely follow Phase II. A recent study in *The New England Journal of Medicine* indicated that nursing mothers on a moderate diet breast-fed successfully while losing weight, and their babies grew and gained weight as expected. The mothers in this study also did moderate exercise, so feel free to add some gentle exercising to your routine. As well, be sure to drink enough fluids, and include three to four servings of low- or non-fat dairy products or calcium-fortified low-fat soy milk.

Obviously, the quality of your food will affect the quality of your breast milk. Remember that many foods, as well as medications, nicotine and alcohol, cross into the breast milk, so don't go crazy with the celebratory champagne. Remind your physician that you are nursing if any new medications are prescribed, and avoid taking over-the-counter drugs. You may notice that certain foods—onions and garlic are notorious—will affect the taste of your breast milk, sometimes upsetting your baby's stomach, too.

Fatigue

Feeling exhausted almost seems to be a chronic condition in new mothers. Gone are the days of looking forward to six to eight hours of continuous sleep; soon four hours of uninterrupted sleep will seem like a luxury! If this is your first child, you can count on getting some rest during the day, when the baby sleeps. But if you have a toddler and a newborn, a daytime nap may be out of the question. This means that diet becomes even more critical for maintaining your energy and health, though the demands of a new baby make it hard to think about cooking or preparing food. For the first few weeks, try to have your partner or a relative cook for you or bring home nutritious takeout. Don't try to be the superwoman; hand over the reins and be grateful for any help. Be sure to have adequate protein at each meal and snack. Adequate iron is crucial, too: this is a good time to eat lean red meat and eggs.

Dear Rick,

I can't believe that after two pregnancies, and at the age of thirty-two, I weigh what I did in high school! It's thanks to the G.I. Diet! I've tried other diets, but this is the one that has changed the way I eat and exercise for life. It has changed my understanding and relationship with food. Some additional positive side effects: no more headaches, no more hunger pains, no more periodic mood swings and "blues," no more heartburn, and greatly diminished symptoms of PMS and menstrual discomfort . . . I read the book, began the G.I. Diet and have lost twenty pounds as well as six inches around my waist . . . I have never felt better, more active and more energetic. What a joy to be able to go on long hikes, canoe trips and bike rides with my husband and feel terrific doing it!

Janine

Try to resist the urge to reach for convenient red-light foods, such as chocolate bars or store-bought muffins, when you're hungry. Your blood sugar will only go up, then plummet, leaving you feeling even more tired and hungry. Instead, keep some green-light snacks on hand, including a supply of green-light muffins in the freezer (perhaps you could prepare them in the weeks before your delivery), which will help tide you over during the early days, when you have little time for shopping and cooking.

Keep a stash of green-light nutrition bars around for emergencies.

Although you feel exhausted, try to avoid caffeine, or limit yourself to one cup a day. The first few weeks with a baby can be tough, but things settle down eventually. Enjoy this wonderful phase of parenthood, where everything your baby needs is something you can so easily provide.

Menopause

Fast-forward now through years of career, homemaking or child-rearing to the next great divide in a woman's life: menopause. From the first hot flash to the last night sweat, menopause can last from five to ten years, so buckle your seat belt—it's a long ride, but not necessarily a rough one. Some women breeze through with no complaints at all. Others have to cope with interrupted sleep, a general "off" feeling, loss of energy and/or libido, and those annoying hot flashes that come out of nowhere and make you want to open every window in the middle of winter.

I'm not going to delve into the pros and cons of hormone replacement therapy (or herbal supplements) here. But I want to point out that one of the side effects of menopause is a drop in your metabolic rate, which is a result of decreased estrogen. What this means—and you will probably gain some weight before you figure this out—is that you need fewer calories to maintain your weight. So if you don't cut back on either your portions or high-calorie foods, or increase your exercise, you will probably put on a few pounds. The worst part is that it all seems to head for the waist, the hips and the thighs. This is because estrogen and progesterone help us maintain that female shape—slim around the waist, curvy at the hips and breasts. But with menopause, we start to move closer to the male pattern, acquiring fat around the middle. Sad but true! The drop in estrogen is also connected to an increased risk for osteoporosis, when the bones thin out and become more fragile (see page 127).

What's to be done? If you're having trouble losing (or the number on the scale keeps going up), start Phase I of the G.I. Diet until you arrive at some weight stability. And keep a food diary: it might be that all the life changes involved in menopause have resulted in some subtle compensation in the food department—more snacks, new treats, bigger portions. Time to keep track of what you really eat, and do what you can to cut back on the high-calorie items. And perhaps the best insurance against being buffeted by menopause is to find some exercise you enjoy and can stick with on a regular basis; try swimming, walking, Pilates, Tai Chi, yoga or just getting off the bus or subway a couple of stops earlier on your way to work. The key is consistency, not intensity.

Hot Flashes/Night Sweats

"Is it just me or is it hot in here?" When you're peeling off your sweater and everyone around you is bundled up, you're probably having one of those surges in your internal thermostat that goes along with menopause. During the day, hot flashes are merely annoying, but at night, accompanied by copious sweating, they can interfere with REM sleep and leave you feeling exhausted, even after a full night's sleep. The sweats and flashes are the result of radical shifts in your levels of estrogen and progesterone, as your body changes gear from the ready-for-reproduction state to a more stable, less cyclical state. Some small adjustments to your diet can help alleviate these symptoms. Keep spicy foods to a minimum, especially in the evening. Avoid alcohol and caffeine. Alcohol can suppress REM sleep, and caffeine is not only a stimulant but also increases your urge to urinate, and you don't need the added pressure of having to get up for the bathroom!

The G.I. Diet is designed to sustain us through all the phases of our life. Women who become family caretakers often forget their own health in their focus on the needs of others. But we need to take care of ourselves for our own sake, first of all, and also for the sake of the people who may depend on us.

Women's Health Concerns

Although we'll be dealing with family health in chapter eleven, we'll address a few conditions here that especially affect women. Although women live longer, we also log more trips to the doctor, and experience more pain and more chronic conditions. So men and women look for different kinds of support from nutrition.

Osteoporosis

This is a condition that generally concerns women past menopause, when the decline in estrogen affects the density of the bones. Women also have smaller bones than men, so this makes us more vulnerable to fragility and fractures. Since estrogen does affect bone strength, many women are tempted to try, or to stay on, hormone replacement therapy (HRT) for the sake of their bones. But since recent research has emerged pointing out the disadvantages of HRT for many women, these risks (a slightly elevated risk of heart disease, stroke and breast cancer) must be weighed against your individual risk for osteoporosis. There are also other medications that are effective ways to treat osteoporosis.

The most significant degree of bone density loss occurs in the first two years after menopause, so this is when it is absolutely critical that you maintain the calcium levels described below. Many doctors recommend bone density tests for women every couple of years after the age of fifty. The first gives you a base-level reading, and then you can monitor how these levels fluctuate. When bones lose density, they become porous and lacy, and fracture more easily. If an ordinary fall results in a broken wrist or ankle, be sure to check your bone density levels.

Although the G.I. Diet will go a long way toward delivering all the calcium you require, you should consider adding a daily multivitamin in order to the meet the 1,500 milligram level for postmenopausal women. Your supplement should also include vitamin D, which is necessary for the absorption of calcium. This vitamin is added to foods such as milk, orange juice and soy milk, and can be acquired from sunshine. In northern countries, however, you can't always count on sunshine delivering enough.

If you are lactose-intolerant, shop for lactose-free items, or take a product such as Lactaid to help with the digestion of dairy products. If that's still a problem, rely on a calcium supplement with vitamin D to meet your requirements.

The other strategy for beating osteoporosis is to make sure you do regular weight-bearing exercise, such as walking or working out with small weights. You need to work your bones! Weight-bearing exercise is also all-round good exercise for your heart and your weight management. And walking is free (unless, of course, you want to invest in a pricey pair of walking shoes, which is a good motivator). If your knees give you trouble or your arches are flat, you might look into orthotics, which give arch support and take some of the pressure off overtaxed knees.

Breast Cancer

Most of us know someone touched by this disease—a sister, a mother, a friend. Or perhaps you have been one of the unlucky one out of nine women who develops breast cancer. The key risk factors include having a mother or sister with breast cancer, early onset of menstruation, or a late first pregnancy. But it can also strike for no clear reason at all. Regardless of your risk factors, diet can play a role in protecting you against this disease.

Recent research has shown that being overweight can increase your chances of developing breast cancer. If you are postmenopausal and overweight, you are at a 30 percent greater risk; if your BMI is in the obesity range, your risk is twice what it is for people of normal weight. It also appears that saturated (bad) fats raise your risk, too. Studies of women living in Japan who get only 10 to 15 percent of their diet from animal fats (i.e., saturated fats) show that they have significantly lower rates of breast cancer than North Americans. But when Japanese women move to North America and switch to a typical North American diet, their breast cancer rates change too, becoming the same as other North American women.

Excess alcohol consumption has also been linked to an increased risk of breast cancer, so the G.I. Diet will help you cut back on that front, too.

Polycystic Ovary Syndrome (PCOS)

Between 5 and 10 percent of women will be diagnosed with polycystic ovary syndrome sometime during their reproductive years. PCOS is a condition associated with insulin resistance, which leads to hyperinsulinemia and often obesity. What this means is that the body's ability to get the sugar out of the blood is defective; the cells are unusually "resistant" to insulin. The pancreas must then secrete more and more insulin to get the sugar out of the blood and into the cells. These high levels of insulin wreak havoc in the body, causing polycystic ovaries, weight gain or difficulty losing weight, increased risk of heart disease and, by age forty, up to a 40 percent increase in the risk of Type 2 diabetes or lack of glucose tolerance.

There is no scientific evidence at this time to say that one specific diet is significantly better than another for PCOS, although studies are underway. But there is some evidence that diets promoting stable blood sugar levels are helpful. As a result, some physicians recommend low-glycemic programs like the G.I. Diet, which is a good choice for anyone at risk for Type 2 diabetes.

Depression

Clinical depression is a multi-faceted disorder, often requiring specific treatment. Often it is genetically determined, passing from one generation to the next. However,

Dear Rick,
I'm eating food I love and still losing weight. All my family have been eating the G.I. Diet way, even though I'm the only one who has to lose weight. I suffer from Polycystic Ovarian Syndrome, which increases insulin resistance, making it harder to lose weight. So the results I'm having are even better. I never thought I would lose the weight this easily.
Emma

between feeling good about ourselves and being clinically depressed lies a whole range of feelings. We often describe ourselves as feeling "depressed" or "down," and this is where diet, and specifically the G.I. Diet, can be helpful. And while the G.I. Diet cannot cure clinical depression, it may help relieve some of the symptoms.

The G.I. Diet helps by stabilizing blood sugar levels, and we know this helps stabilize mood. When a person is depressed, blood levels of the mood-regulating neuro-transmitter serotonin are lower than normal. Carbohydrates temporarily raise serotonin levels, which is why we reach for high-G.I., simple-carb "comfort foods" such as dough-nuts, bagels and cookies. And as we know, simple carbs boost our blood sugar levels quickly, and just as quickly they fall again. And so does our mood. Complex carbs help stabilize our serotonin levels and mood without spiking our blood sugar levels.

Being overweight can be depressing and bad for self-esteem. Attempting diets and failing can often add to these feelings of depression. And with so many fad diets out there promising miracles, failure is almost inevitable. The G.I. Diet may produce a less dramatic rate of weight loss, but the weight is more likely to stay off. And as so many of our readers tell us, self-confidence and feeling good accompany that permanent weight loss.

Finally, research has shown that regular exercise can relieve symptoms of depression—another reason to put on those sneakers and get walking.

TO SUM UP

Women need:

- enough iron to make up for loss through menstruation
- an "anti-PMS" diet that promotes stable blood sugar levels
- sufficient body fat to ensure a healthy reproductive system
- enough calcium for child-bearing and to inhibit the development of osteoporosis after menopause
- careful attention to diet during pregnancy and breast-feeding to sustain a healthy baby
- a diet low in saturated fat
- a diet with a low glycemic index

CHAPTER EIGHT

Getting Your Partner on Deck

Let's say you live with someone who is indifferent to diets and perfectly happy with how the family currently eats. But you aren't. You may want to lose weight yourself, and you don't want to do double duty in the kitchen, cooking one meal for yourself and another for everyone else. You may be concerned about your partner's weight more than your own; or you might want your partner to help you turn the children's eating habits around.

How do you get your unmotivated partner to go along with the G.I. Diet?

First, figure out if your partner wants to—or should— lose weight. Since over half the population is overweight, chances are he or she has a pound or two to lose. In the last chapter, Ruth talked about the issues specific to women that affect their weight and health. Now let's look at the issues that are specific to men.

Men have more muscle mass than women, and muscle

burns a lot of calories. As we mentioned earlier, we all start to lose muscle mass after our twenties. This process accelerates after forty in women, and for men it steps up after sixty. But since men's total muscle loss is greater than it is for women, this has more influence on their weight, because they're using far fewer calories than when they were younger. For men, this is what suddenly puts the weight on in middle age. Also, with careers peaking and more family obligations, men may not be playing sports or exercising as much as they did when they were younger.

A second factor is alcohol. Men drink twice as much as women, and there are three times as many heavy drinkers among men than women. Alcohol is packed with calories and sits at the top of the G.I. red-light charts. "Beer belly" says it all.

The third factor is body image. Men simply don't obsess about this in the same way many women do. Being a few pounds up or down—or even many pounds—doesn't necessarily concern them. We all know big, out-of-shape men who don't feel their sex appeal is compromised in the least. Women, on the other hand, can become slaves to body image, never satisfied with their weight or how they look. Whether men are masters of denial or simply lack a woman's finely tuned body awareness, it certainly makes it easier for them to ignore diet and nutrition issues. So if they aren't driven by a desire to get back into their 34-inch pants, what *is* going to motivate them to join you on the G.I. Diet?

Well, fear of dying might get their attention. If your partner really needs to lose some weight, enlist his doctor's help. Let a doctor tell him about the connection between excess weight and diabetes, heart disease, stroke and cancer. Does he know the link between the saturated fats in porterhouse steaks and the health of his prostate? Is he aware of the association between weight, hypertension and dying of a stroke? If vanity isn't the main issue with many men in terms of losing weight, fear of ill health or of dropping dead at fifty-eight of a heart attack might work.

Males appear to be at greater risk than women for heart disease, stroke and colon cancer. These are all major killers among men. Prostate cancer now kills nearly the same number of men as breast cancer does women. All these conditions are significantly affected by weight and the nature of your diet.

Now get out the tape measure. If your husband's waist measurement is more than 40 inches, he is putting his health in jeopardy. Does he want to miss seeing his children growing up? Do you want to lose your mate and carry the burden of family alone? OK, these are nasty scare tactics, but they are also based on medical reality.

Besides, men want to feel slim and look young too, even if they don't wring their hands about it the way women do. And as soon as they see (and feel) the benefits of losing weight, they won't have to be convinced.

But what if giving up the after-work beer is unthinkable? What if his mother brought him up on giant portions of lasagna and he can't imagine life without it? Scolding and bossing, as you may have discovered, don't work. The best way to change your partner's eating habits is to stock the house with green-light foods and to provide appealing green-light alternatives to his red-light regulars. Here are some of the recipes you will find in part three that turn traditional meals into green-light ones: Open-Faced Meatball Subs, Mushroom and Gravy Pork Chops, Chicken Fried Rice and Apple Raspberry Coffee Cake.

Once your partner realizes that the G.I. Diet isn't just "rabbit food" and deprivation, that he can eat often, lose weight and not go hungry, you may be surprised at how easily he'll be converted. If he notices that he feels more energetic and that the after-dinner slump has disappeared, he'll realize that this way of eating delivers rewards, both short-term and long-term.

But perhaps you live with a hard-core objector. He'll eat tuna salad at home, then hit the Wendy's drive-through on the way to the ball game. Or he'll go along with the food part as long as he can keep up the cocktails and wine.

There are two routes available in this case. One is to leave him alone. You take the G.I. Diet route and let your partner watch your transformation into a slimmer, more energetic, healthier person. Let him notice people noticing how good you look. Once he sees the rewards of the diet—physical and social—he may feel more like joining you.

Or you can always try the stealth method. Don't try a hard sell. Simply change the family's menu and say nothing. A friend of mine who went on the G.I. Diet began serving herself and her husband green-light meals for dinner every night, without telling him they were G.I. He wasn't aware he was on a weight-loss program until he had to buy a new belt!

If you and your partner are raising kids, you should both be aware of what example you're setting: is it the Homer Simpson diet (I'll have twice what he's having) or an attitude toward food that includes weight control, good nutrition, enjoyment of eating and prevention of disease?

If you are a divorced dad sharing the parental duties with your ex, don't succumb to the stereotype of the fast-food dad dining in restaurants with his weekend brood. Show your kids that eating together, preparing meals together and making dinner a family occasion is not going to stop. And don't say you love them with endless treats. Show them you care about them by caring *for* them, through their diet and nutrition. The G.I. Diet is a simple way to organize your single-parent game plan. All you have to do is follow the traffic-light charts.

TO SUM UP

Having your spouse/partner involved is important because:

- It makes shopping and food preparation easier.
- It provides you with mutual support and encouragement.
- It represents a cohesive and united front as role models for the family.
- Even if weight loss is not an issue, health will improve through eating better.

CHAPTER NINE

Are Your Kids Eating Well?

Food and children: it couldn't be more important, and it couldn't be more emotionally charged as well. What your children eat has an impact on every aspect of their lives: behaviour, mood, energy, concentration, performance in school and vulnerability to infection and disease. Food is also a source of pleasure and at the centre of family gatherings and celebrations. It's a popular source of conflict, too! Getting a handle on mealtimes is often half the battle in making the whole family run smoothly.

Food also plays an important role in managing medical disorders, including allergies, asthma (which can be related to food allergies) and attention deficit hyperactivity disorder (ADHD). ADHD affects about 4 percent of the population and has been linked to childhood obesity. Drugs have been the first line of treatment, but changes in diet can also help.

Then there is the weight issue. According to Statistics

Canada, about 37 percent of children aged two to eleven are overweight, and 8 percent of them are obese. As health reporter Andre Picard wrote in *The Globe and Mail* (May 2005) on the subject of this shocking modern epidemic of overweight kids: "Children do not want to be fat. When they are, they pay a terrible price. For the most part, they are voiceless in this discussion and powerless victims of an underlying phenomenon. Overweight and obese children are the product of modern society, one that is characterized by an environment where we have engineered activity out of daily life and adopted a lifestyle that has seen us transform our food into a chemical smorgasbord of fats and sugars wolfed down on the run."

How do we begin to address all these concerns? The G.I. Diet offers one way to turn your family eating habits around. Rich in fruit, vegetables, whole grains, low-fat dairy products and meat, nuts and legumes, the G.I. Diet is ideal for growing children. In this chapter, we'll explore ways to involve your children in eating the green-light way, and how to adapt the diet to children with a weight problem, whether they are over- or underweight. **Note: This chapter does not apply to children under two and a half years; they have specific nutritional needs. For guidelines about feeding your baby, consult your doctor.**

The G.I. Diet and Children

Changing what your family eats is easier said than done! What if your children are perfectly happy living in the no-vegetable zone, on a diet of pizza pockets, Kraft Dinner and Choco-Slams? You are probably going to meet some resistance as you try to steer the family meals in a healthier direction. Kids are conservative in their appetites. All the love and goodwill in the world are sometimes not enough to get a ten-year-old to try grilled halibut with mango salsa for the first time. And pushing a new approach to food is often complicated by family dynamics, which tend to play out during mealtimes. This can create tension around who eats what and how much. As many parents have learned, eating is also the area where children can first express their autonomy and exert control—by spitting out that avocado or clamping their mouths shut. So it's all too easy for food to become a nasty power issue, with parents and kids on opposite teams.

Mothers especially can invest too much emotion in what their children eat: to feed them, after all, is to love them. To love them even more is to give them more food. Treats can become a way to compensate for not having enough time to spend with your kids. As a result of all these emotional currents, mealtime can be fraught with good intentions and bad eating behaviour.

So as the parent, remember that you are the pivotal factor in how and what your children eat. More often than not, it's up to the mother to decide what everyone in the family eats at home. But it's not just about making the right sort of grocery list; it's also about the attitude that you and your partner share—or don't share—toward food choices, weight, body image and eating. Food is so personal! Perhaps your husband grew up in a family that believed no dinner was complete without 8 or 10 ounces of red meat and a rich dessert. Maybe you had a strict father who made you sit at the table until the last lima bean on your plate was eaten. Now, to your horror, you find yourself doing exactly the same thing with your own child: using food as punishment. Or you might react to too many food rules by doing the opposite with your own children: setting no boundaries at all when it comes to food.

As parents, we need to be vigilant that we are not passing on the poor eating behaviours and attitudes toward weight that we may have grown up with. These only increase the chances of our children developing eating disorders or their own problems with weight control. Where food is concerned, the sins of the father (and mother) are truly visited on their children.

These cycles must be broken if we want to do something about the wave of childhood obesity in our culture. The first and simplest way to change, however, is not to add new rules but to lighten up around food. Don't try to overmanage or control how much or what your child eats. Instead, learn to trust your child. Believe it or not, children *will* eat and are quite capable of regulating their food intake. They want to survive after all. And their bodies are good at telling them what they need to survive. Yes, they might refuse to try new foods at first; this aversion stems from primitive times, when experimenting with new foods or unknown plants could turn out to be fatal. Reassure them that tofu is not, in fact, going to kill them. But don't force it on them. Instead, make new food choices part of mealtimes, so they can experiment or not. Make something different for yourself and let them see you enjoying it. What's important is the kind of "food environment" you create for them in the home—keeping nutritious things handy and getting rid of the junk food. Then let your children come round to new foods in their own good time. In fact, the more you try to cajole or force food on children, the more likely they are to develop a resistance to eating.

Pushing food is one problem; refusing to let them have any of their favourite foods is another fast route to failure. Too many restrictions in the home may make children overeat when they're out with their friends. So give up on total control. Step back, relax, focus on positive parenting instead, and take a good look at your own eating habits first.

Are you a yo-yo dieter, swinging from a few weeks of rigid rules to an anything-goes attitude? Are you an "emotional eater," taking comfort in double-fudge ice cream at the end of a bad day? Is your husband a breakfast skipper or a potato-chips-and-TV snacker? If yes, then you can't expect your son to sit beside the two of you with a dish of carrot sticks and a whole wheat cracker. The way you relate to food yourself will have the greatest impact on your children's relationship to food. To change them, you have to change yourself as well.

The basic framework governing the relationships between you, your child and food depends on clearly defined roles and responsibilities for both parent and child. Ellyn Slater, in her excellent book *How to Get Your Kid to Eat . . . but Not Too Much,* suggests a simple formula to prevent food from becoming a battleground:

1. You are the role model who is responsible for *providing meals,* as well as *when* and *where* they will be served.
2. Your children are responsible for *what* and *how much* they eat.

In other words, it's what you do, not what you say, that counts. If you doubt this, think about your mother's feelings around food and ask yourself how it has affected you or your siblings. Maybe she got angry when people were late coming to the table. Do you get upset when people take their time showing up for dinner?

Where do you begin to change your family's eating habits? First of all, if you have been in the habit of catering to different appetites, let your family know that everyone will now be eating the same main meals. No more short-order cooking. No more grabbing things out of the fridge at all hours. It means that the family will eat together at set times. Maybe not every night at six o'clock—lessons, practices and social lives often interfere—but schedule meals in a consistent and regular pattern. For instance, on Monday,

Wednesday and Friday, your kids can expect a meal on the table at a certain time and they are expected to be there, too.

It also means that eating together should be a light-hearted time. Keep it enjoyable. This is how we foster a positive attitude toward nutrition and sharing. Don't use meals as an opportunity to raise family problems and conflicts. Not that we're trying to recreate *Father Knows Best* here, with the fifties-style nuclear family—mother in the kitchen, wearing pearls and heels with her shirtwaist dress, and her two well-scrubbed boys sitting at the table. That was probably a fantasy even then! What we are trying to establish is a little *structure* and *predictability* regarding family meals. Believe it or not, most children look for and are grateful for some order and coherence in our uncertain world.

Let's look a little more closely at what's involved if you want to initiate your family into the G.I. way of eating.

How Are You With Food?

It's fine to talk the talk—but when it comes to getting your kids to eat more healthily, you have to walk the walk. What, when and how much you eat is going to influence your children much more than a weekly lecture on eating more fresh fruit. Recent research in the U.S. found that girls who don't like to try new foods are likely to have moms who don't eat a variety of foods, especially vegetables. Try to remember: your grandchildren are probably

Dear Rick,

My six-year-old son (without any encouragement from me) has begun to change his eating habits after watching what I now eat. Although I am fairly careful with what I feed to him at main meals, his lunchtime sandwich fillings have always been fairly plain and unimaginative (by his choice). But now, for example, he is requesting sandwiches consisting of no less than cucumber, carrot, shaved chicken breast, baby spinach leaves, arugula, tomato and cheese. What's even better is that he makes it himself and takes great pleasure in eating his own creation. So not only has your book changed my life, but it's shaping the future for my son's eating habits as well.

Thank you,

Tania

going to have a few of your eating habits, so make them good ones.

When I was growing up in the U.K., we rarely ate fish at home, except for the traditional fried fish and chips, brought home wrapped in newspaper. So I decided I didn't like fish. When I was raising my own family, my eldest son picked up on this and decided he didn't like fish either. Then I made a conscious effort to change my eating habits and discovered the delights of fresh fish and seafood. We now eat seafood at least twice a week, and our grown-up children have become seafood enthusiasts, too.

A change for the better is welcome, but it also helps to be consistent in what you eat. If you have an all-pizza week, followed by a zero-carb diet week, your children aren't going to listen when you say it's important to drink milk every single day. And children *like* predictability. They have no problem with the idea that if it's Friday, it's going to be fish. But if your own eating is feast one day, famine the next, or full of guilt over indulging in the "wrong things," then your children's approach to food will be erratic or fraught with "issues," too.

Mothers should think twice before they burden their daughters and sons with conversations about being too fat. If you have a thing about your thighs, try not to confide in your eleven-year-old daughter about your fixation. Let children feel good about who they are, regardless of what they weigh—and especially if they need to lose weight. The culture is already hard enough on girls and weight without your "weighing in" with negative remarks that only reinforce this anxiety around having the right sort of curves.

It's more effective to point out the positive results of eating a better diet—the extra energy, the optimism, the social confidence of no longer being overweight, and the feeling of doing the right thing for your body and your health. Don't scare kids into losing weight. It will only backfire in the end.

And don't set up your partner as a bad example either. "Your mother needs to lose weight, so we're all on a diet" is not going to inspire anyone. Kids don't like to hear one parent being disparaged by another. Try to get your partner onside, so he doesn't look down at his G.I. plate with its one corner of whole wheat pasta and say, "That's not real pasta!" If both of you are enthusiastic about eating the green-light way, your kids are already halfway there. You don't want your partner winking at his son and saying, "Eat your salad, then I'll take you out for a McFlurry."

Involving the Family in Shopping and Preparation

Children are often excluded from food shopping, meal planning and food preparation. There's no reason for this, except that parents are usually rushed and don't want to further complicate their chores. But getting your kids involved in shopping the green-light way is a great strategy for making them feel more in charge of what they eat. And they will learn about nutrition along the way. So engage your kids in this new eating venture. Make it their project, too.

Rather than focus on weight management, talk about this as something that's going to make life better in all kinds of ways—energy, health, appearance, vitality. Explain that it won't be a temporary trial run either. This is how you're going to eat from now on. But don't try to oversell it to your family. You can just consult the traffic-light colour charts, make a list and start shopping.

With your older kids, show them the food charts. You'll be amazed by how quickly they will adopt the traffic-light system and make it part of their language. Many of you will remember the small voice in the back seat telling you to buckle up when seat belts were first made mandatory. This time, it'll be "Is that chocolate doughnut green-light, Mom?"

If they can read, assign them "hunting expeditions" in the supermarket: can they find the whole wheat penne? A canned soup with three kinds of beans in it? Which low-fat yogurt is their favourite? Can they find the one with sucralose in it, not aspartame? It's a scavenger hunt for green-light food. Showing kids how to decipher food labels will stand them in good stead for the rest of their lives.

Involve them in the kitchen, too. Our three boys used to help prepare our green-light snacks, such as muffins (see pages 274–77 for the recipes). We have photos of these early bakers, complete with their long aprons and large wooden spoons. Children are usually more enthusiastic about what they eat if they helped cook it themselves. Younger children can always wash vegetables, fill measuring cups, stir ingredients or set the table. The older ones can make simple recipes like scrambled eggs, oatmeal cookies and pancakes. Encourage your teenagers to take over the cooking for one family meal a week, if they enjoy working in the kitchen. Let them concoct whatever they want, as long as it fits the green-light guidelines, then give them lots of applause and recognition for a job well done.

Food should be an integral part of family life regardless of what sort of family you have, not just something one parent takes charge of. If your partner doesn't want to cook, ask him to at least play some role in the food department, such as shopping, grilling or growing herbs in the garden. If you're a single mother, resist the temptation of drive-through fast food for you and your kids on your way home from hockey practice. If you're a single father who puts dinner on the table every night, congratulations. Your kids will thank you later (even if they hate the idea of zucchini now).

The Importance of Regular Mealtimes

When the whole family is on a regular schedule—school, daycare, work, then home again—it's easier to structure mealtimes. But during the summer or on weekends, the whole family can get into all-day snacking and grazing, which is disastrous for weight control and exasperating for the family cook. One minute you're scrambling eggs for the youngest, the next you're putting frozen pizza in the oven for the older ones. Once your children learn that you are willing to play short-order cook, you might as well give up!

So set clear, firm times when meals and snacks will be served. If they miss out, too bad. Make a big pot of cooked oatmeal in the morning, and try to make sure everyone sits down to a bowl of it, with fruit and skim milk. It takes five extra minutes. It might be harder with your teenager. They're notorious for sleeping in, then running out the door and skipping breakfast, or eating a cereal bar on the run. At least make breakfast available to them. Then they might take the two minutes to eat it.

If it's summer or the weekend and everyone's in and out of the house, set snack times as well as a dinner hour. At 4 p.m., they can help themselves to the low-fat yogurt or fruit or green-light muffins in the fridge. Otherwise, the fridge stays shut. Grazing all day long encourages high-fat, highly processed, high-calorie choices, and makes it hard to keep track of what you've eaten. So reaching into the fridge for a hunk of cheese is not encouraged. The idea is to sit down together to eat on a regular basis, and at the same time, as often as possible.

The Family Dinner Hour

This is an endangered activity. Fewer and fewer families actually sit down together to a cooked meal. Instead, they bring home fast food and eat in front of the TV. This is fun once in a blue moon, but not as a steady diet. Research has shown that people who watch TV while eating tend to overeat. Or another familiar scenario: the family cook prepares a "kids'" meal, then when the spouse gets home from work, they sit down to "adult" food while the kids do homework or watch television.

But eating together not only lets you have more control over nutrition, it fosters many good things: enjoying each other's company, developing manners, conversation and trying new kinds of food. Naturally, people come to the table in all sorts of moods: tired, wound up or angry at a sibling across the table who likes to fight. The dinner table doesn't have to be all peace and harmony, but that time together should be there. Don't talk about family problems. Do that away from the table. Instead, make it a time that is about enjoying the food on the table and each other's company. Younger kids may not want to stay in their chairs too long. Fine. They can manage the main course at least. Just serve a variety of healthy food and let them try it, reject it or simply watch you enjoy it. Exposing them to good food is all you need to do at first.

And, if possible, create a pleasing environment. Set the table nicely. Turn off the TV, the video games and the cellphones. Eat slowly. It takes at least twenty to thirty minutes for the "I'm full" message to get from stomach to brain.

But again, don't be too rigid around the rules. If there is one night when everyone wants to watch something on TV, at least watch and eat together, and maybe talk about it, too!

Pay attention to the serving portions. In our supersized environment, we tend to offer unnecessarily large portions, even to children. If someone is only 25 percent of your body weight, don't serve them 75 percent of your portion. The best solution is to serve foods such as pasta and vegetables in large bowls and have everyone help themselves. Show them how to judge portions by how much of the plate each food covers, remembering that pasta or potatoes should only cover a quarter of the plate and vegetables can fill half the plate. Portions of meat or fish should be the size of the palm of your hand, or a quarter of their plate. Serving themselves helps children take charge of what they eat.

Let's look at other ways that children can learn to eat well.

Getting Children to Love the Right Kind of Food

"Just one more bite!" "Here comes the plane into the hangar." "Look, I made this especially for you." Do these sound familiar? My mother's favourite, which she still uses at the age of ninety-five, is "I love to see an empty plate!" My father liked to "fly" fingers of toast dipped in egg yolk into the mouths of his grandchildren, with all the appropriate aircraft sounds. And then there's the least effective form of persuasion: "Remember the starving children in Africa." How is that supposed to get kids to eat more than they want to?

So cajoling doesn't work, and bribery is not a good idea either. Using treats such as dessert or candy as a reward only reinforces the appeal of the wrong kind of foods. Forcing children to stay at the table until they've finished what's on the plate is ineffective, too. Associating food with punishment is hardly going to encourage healthy eating habits!

I'm Not Hungry

But if you eliminate coaxing, bribing and scolding, how *do* you get kids to eat? What if you cook the world's best grilled tuna salad, with snow peas and lovely boiled new potatoes, and your child glares at his plate and announces, "I'm not hungry." Fine. Let them know they don't have to eat if they don't want to, but they have to stay at the table and keep the family company. And make it clear you're not going to rustle up something else for them an hour later either. Meals and snacks happen at set times. These are the ground rules. You'll find that hunger is a great motivator. You might also be surprised at how quickly they adapt to a firm schedule around eating.

The Broccoli Challenge

Kids, as I mentioned, don't like to try new things, especially vegetables. Things like kale or Swiss chard or other green veggies often have a slightly bitter taste; in evolutionary terms, people were reluctant to try new things in case they were poison, and bitterness was often associated with poisonous foods. Breast milk, on the other hand, has a sweetish taste. Perhaps that's one reason why smooth, sweet things appeal to kids so much.

But childhood is about exploring and experimenting, which is what growing up is all about. And that goes for food as well. So be adventurous with nutritious food and with the occasional treats as well. Try the no-sugar licorice frozen yogurt. Buy oatmeal raisin cookies for a change.

And explore exotic fruits—blackberries, guavas, asian pears, mandarin oranges. Just as children acquire language skills and reading fluency, they should also develop a knowledge and taste for a wide variety of foods.

Researchers claim that it takes ten to fifteen exposures to a new food before it's fully accepted. If your children don't like the texture of whole wheat pasta compared with the white flour variety, try it again the following week, with a different sauce. They'll get used to it, just as our family got used to skim milk instead of 2% or whole milk.

As for snacks, low-fat yogurts now come in a host of different sizes and flavours, and most kids take to them quickly. Vegetable sticks are great snacks to serve fresh with a yogurt-based dip or hummus. We always kept a plate of sliced or baby carrots, celery sticks and sweet pepper slices in the fridge for the boys. If it's prepared and handy, they will eat it, especially if there aren't any brownies beside them. To this day, veg and dip is a favourite snack in our family.

So the trick to introducing new foods is to offer them without pushing, and to just keep offering them without pushing. I still hate cooked spinach, ever since I was "obliged" to eat it as a child.

Eating should be fun. Make your mealtimes light-hearted; the concrete benefits of weight loss and better nutrition will follow. Encourage kids to develop a sense of accountability and responsibility by making their own choices just as grown-ups do.

Every stage of childhood has different challenges when it comes to diet. Let's look at each of them in more detail.

Toddler/Preschool

The years from two to five are the time when children are most resistant to new foods, especially fresh vegetables. This is when they learn the power of "no" and of rejecting food.

Some parents find that if they introduce different kinds of puréed vegetables when first adding solids to their baby's diet, he or she will develop a liking for things like squash, pumpkin, spinach and broccoli. But when a two-year-old doesn't enjoy the taste of something, he usually lets you know in no uncertain terms! Most of us can remember the first time our toddlers dumped a dish of peas on the floor or spit out a spoonful of egg. Texture is important, too. Sometimes mushed carrots won't appeal, but (when they reach chewing age) carrot sticks with a cup of yogurt for dipping will. Even the shape of the food can make a difference. Celery with hummus in the groove is more fun than plain carrot sticks.

The best way to help your kids open up to new foods is to include them on outings to the supermarket and to restaurants. But let's face facts: as parents of a small child, you are probably going to spend more time at Tim Hortons than in fancy restaurants. In that case, steer your child away from the sugary foods, toward the things that still qualify as green-light: meat-and-bean chili, a roast turkey sandwich on whole wheat, a low-fat yogurt parfait with berries. Although advertising and peer pressure are hard to counter, it is possible to raise your toddler to really enjoy fresh vegetables and unprocessed, unpackaged food. It's all a matter of teaching their palette to enjoy different tastes, in the same way you would read to them from many kinds of books or make sure they visit parks as well as museums. An education in food is as important as any other kind of learning.

From Five to Twelve

These are the years when children develop passionate attachments to certain foods and a shuddering revulsion toward others. You will know by now whether your child is a food adventurer or someone who would live only on hot dogs if you let him. I know one boy who grew up in a family of superb cooks, and he was a hot dog aficionado. His mother worried, but eventually he branched out—and he survived.

When kids start school, they are also going to be eating lunch with friends and having sleepovers where a bucket of chicken nuggets is the big draw. The way to balance this school-age romance with fast food and sugary cereals is to calmly let it happen; at the same time, make sure what they eat at home is nutritious and varied. Adopt the 75 percent rule:

THE 75 PERCENT SOLUTION

The golden rule with children, as with adults on the G.I. Diet, is not to turn it into a straitjacket. As we wrote earlier, if you keep to the G.I. Diet 90 percent of the time, you'll do well. It's important to give yourself a little leeway for those inevitable situations where you can't control what you eat. And children need more leeway — 75 percent — to allow for the influence of peer pressure and simple experimentation. Kids don't want to be the only ones bringing a Thermos of black bean soup to school, even if they secretly love it. Let them eat what their friends like to eat some of the time. Just keep the home fare green-light and add in yellow-light foods if weight is not an issue. If you can pack green- and yellow-light lunches 75 percent of the time, you'll be ahead of the game, and your kids won't resent your attitude toward food.

Teenage Boys and Girls

So much goes on between the ages of twelve and twenty: puberty, explosive physical growth, the testing of family bonds and independence, the development of a social network that counts as much (if not more) than the family circle, not to mention the possibility of falling in love and discovering sexual expression. No wonder it's an intense, exasperating and bewildering time for parents as well.

What role does food and diet play in the midst of these roller-coaster years? First of all, it provides nutrition for one of the most important stages in your children's physical growth. Second, it expresses your love for them, even during difficult times. And third, it establishes a relationship with food they will take with them into adulthood. Even when your teenager doesn't want to talk to you about a broken heart, she will probably say yes to homemade muffins.

Adolescence is also when food portions either explode or radically shrink. Unfortunately, there is a gender side to all this: teenage boys can develop enormous appetites, while teenage girls, driven by body image concerns, can try to diet in all kinds of unwise ways, which may undermine their nutrition. Your son might think that a mixing bowl full of Cheerios is the answer to his big appetite, but there are other solutions. And your teenage daughter needs to know that not eating is the *worst* way to lose weight. She'll only gain it right back. Show her yourself that eating more green-light kinds of food will keep her from yo-yoing between extremes of starvation and indulgence. Research indicates that yo-yo dieters end up putting on even more weight than they initially lost! The ideal is slow, steady weight loss or maintaining a stable weight.

If your daughter says she wants to lose weight, check to see if her concern is valid by determining her BMI with the information in appendix IV on page 300. If her BMI indicates that she is overweight, give her *The G.I. Diet* to read. Then let her be in charge of selecting the green-light foods she prefers. Make sure she includes good sources of iron, either in food (dark green leafy vegetables, for instance) or through a supplement. Menstruating girls need more iron. Help them set reasonable, achievable limits. In order to avoid playing food cop, purge the pantry of tempting red-light items that you or your partner may want to keep around.

Also, remind your kids that everyone is blessed with a different body type and metabolism, and that there is no universal ideal when it comes to weight.

If your daughter is not overweight, then emphasize that sound nutrition is more valuable than struggling to make it down to size zero. Naturally, the cultural environment plays a big role in our attitudes toward fat and thin. Advertising images, rock stars and fashion have a profound influence on how teenagers want to look. But it may not be enough to encourage your children to look beyond trends and television. Unfortunately, adolescence is also a time when eating disorders take hold, especially among teenage girls. The most familiar ones are anorexia nervosa, when they refuse food or eat very little, and bulimia, when they binge on food, then purge through vomiting. Anorexia can be serious, even fatal; when body weight drops below a certain critical point, organs become damaged and can fail. Bulimia can be disastrous to health as well; even teeth enamel suffers from the acidic effect of constant purging.

Pay attention to extreme dieting or weight loss in your adolescent daughter. The best way to approach an eating disorder is with your unconditional support and love, along with good professional help. We may never get to the bottom of the whys of eating disorders, but we can certainly help prevent them by encouraging a relaxed and positive attitude toward eating.

If, as parents, you are having a rough ride with your adolescent children, one way to offer stability and love is to stick to a regular schedule of family meals and to keep the fridge stocked with green- and yellow-light foods—with room left over for a few totally red-light items that they can't live without. If you can lighten up on the food front while making sure that good food is always handy in the house, you will create an environment that supports and nourishes in every sense.

Skipping meals is common among teenagers. A third of teenage girls, one study estimated, regularly skip breakfast. Since their bodies are in the process of doubling in weight, sleep is at a premium, and sleeping in often becomes more important than sitting down to breakfast in the morning. This starts the domino effect of plunging blood sugar, followed by something sweet to give them energy, and maybe a day of snacks that ends with them overeating at dinner. This is the perfect formula for the classic hyperglycemic/hypoglycemic yo-yo, in which they bounce from high to low blood sugar, with the accompanying fatigue and mood swings. Since everything else in their lives is changing so radically, it's a good idea to at least try to keep the blood sugar stable!

The skipping-breakfast routine has also been linked to being overweight. A recent Oxford University study compared two groups of school-age children. One group ate a high-G.I. breakfast, the other a low-G.I. one. At lunch, they were free to choose and eat as much as they wanted. Those on the high-G.I. breakfast ate considerably more than those who had the low-G.I. fare. The facts speak for themselves. But practically speaking, how do you convince your headstrong teenager not to bolt out the door with nothing but a chocolate bar in his pocket? Well, if he won't sit down, at least equip him with a green-light-version nutrition bar, in which the fat and sugar content is as low as possible. Better yet, prepare old-fashioned oatmeal for breakfast. Serve it with blueberries, walnuts, unsweetened applesauce—whatever strange combinations of green-light toppings he may enjoy. If it's ready when he passes through the kitchen, it will take him two minutes to down it, and it will steady his boat for the rest of the day. You might have to get him on the breakfast program with something more appealing at first, like a fried back-bacon sandwich. But once he compares how he feels on a no-breakfast morning to a day he begins with oatmeal or some other green-light food, he may see the light.

The other way to promote healthy eating and curb peer pressure to eat junk is to encourage your kids to have their friends over and entertain. Mix up your green- and yellow-light food with a few red-light favourites. Let them enjoy offering food and making up their own food combinations. Let food choice become part of their growing independence while you keep the shopping and meals green-light.

Dear Rick,
As a teenager, I know that dieting is a big thing for a lot of us. We're always trying different diets to lose the weight. So many of my friends usually end up going hungry. Because I've witnessed this happen so many times, the idea of dieting completely turned me off, until I found your diet. Considering the G.I. Diet was the first diet I've really ever done, I'm surprised that it actually worked. I've managed to lose twenty-four pounds in a healthy, natural way. Even my doctor was pleased. And trust me, I'm never hungry! I don't want to give away my secret to my friends!
Erika

Vegetarians and Vegans

Adolescence is a time when concerns around environmental issues or the treatment of animals can come into play. If your teenager decides to become a vegetarian (eliminating meat from her diet) or a vegan (avoiding all animal products, including eggs and milk), how do you make sure she is getting proper nutrition? How do you shop and cook for a vegan when your husband is a steak lover and your other child won't eat pasta? Well, it's not easy, but it can be done!

Vegetarian eating is more easily accommodated than

veganism, and it has the advantage of emphasizing many foods that are green-light anyway: fresh vegetables, whole grains and beans. Vegetarian diets are closer to the G.I. way of eating than an average diet heavy in processed, sugary or high-fat food. Some teenagers just want to eliminate eating red meat while still enjoying fish, seafood, eggs and other good sources of protein. If this means they will eat more vegetables and whole foods, then the loss of saturated fat in red meat will be a good loss, and getting enough protein won't be a problem if you include nuts, beans, tofu, soy milk and vegetables in their diet. The only vital nutrient you can't obtain from a diet of plant food alone is vitamin B12, and if your child eats dairy products or eggs, she will get enough. What's just as important is iron, but this is available in eggs as well as from dark green leafy vegetables. Vitamin C is important for iron absorption, so it's a good idea to eat oranges or broccoli with iron-rich foods.

The upside of a vegetarian diet—and it is estimated that up to 35 percent of teenagers are trying to eliminate red meat from their diet—is the increased awareness of food. If they are concerned about the quality and the origin of what they eat, they will become more aware of other aspects of eating, too. This is better than food oblivion!

Veganism is a stricter regime, eliminating food from any animal source. So eggs, milk and cheese are out, along with red meat, poultry and seafood. Veganism tends to require more food preparation and careful shopping. This is tougher to integrate into family meals. If your teenager opts for veganism, encourage him to get involved in the cooking and preparation of the meals—you will be grateful for the help. But don't be overly concerned about the nutritional deficits of such a diet. A teenager's protein requirement can be completely met by a diet that includes the following elements daily: 1 cup oatmeal, 1 cup soy milk, 2 slices whole wheat bread, 1 bagel, 2 tbsp peanut butter, 1 cup vegetarian baked beans, 5 oz tofu, 2 tbsp almonds, 1 cup broccoli and 1 cup brown rice.

We tend to overestimate our protein requirements and underestimate the amount of protein contained in whole foods such as grains, potatoes and dried beans. The one concern regarding teenagers and vegetarian diets is the overall amount of calories. They require enough calories to maintain their weight, or to lose weight gradually if that's their goal. So make sure their vegetarian diet is varied. You might need to include certain red- or yellow-light items such as peanut butter, since it's such a popular source of protein; but stick to the natural, all-peanut variety, not sweetened commercial brands.

The only caution with veganism is that this diet does require some form of additional Vitamin B12, which you can get from taking nutritional yeast or a vitamin supplement.

Fast Food and Kids

The fast-food industry has a lot to account for when it comes to our children's nutrition. Most hamburgers, french fries and other fast-food staples are loaded with saturated fat and calories. Then they made it worse by supersizing everything. You can now buy a 72-ounce Pepsi—but why would you? The book *Fast Food Nation* by Eric Schlosser is an eye opener on the subject. You might also have a family viewing of the documentary film *Super Size Me,* by Morgan Spurlock (a book version is available now, too). The filmmaker lived on nothing but McDonald's food three times a day for a month, with devastating effects on his weight and health. His doctor finally told him to stop with the Double Quarter Pounders With Cheese if he valued his liver! It's an entertaining portrait that reveals the poverty and perils of a diet dominated by fast food. (And it caused McDonald's to retire the term "supersize," replacing it with "large.")

But let's face facts: kids are going to eat fast food from time to time, and your family is going to wind up eating at McDonald's or Burger King now and then. For suggestions on navigating their menus, see the Fast Food section on pages 70–76. With all the red-light temptations, my best advice is to keep family visits to fast-food restaurants to a minimum.

The one exception to the fast-food fat gauntlet is the Subway chain. It provides an excellent range of green-light options, many with less than 7 grams of fat. Just avoid the Atkins-style wraps, which feature turkey, bacon and sauce; they taste great but are absolutely loaded with saturated fat and calories. The best solution to eating out is to choose family restaurants.

Lunches

This can be tricky. School cafeterias vary from one community to another, and some offer questionable nutritional choices. The only way to have some control over this is to raise your voice and let your school board know your concerns regarding food.

Your other option is to pack a lunch for your children, regardless of how old they are. This chore might be more efficient if you organize your own lunches along with your children's, so only one prep session is required for the whole family. There are tips for turning your child's brown bag into a green-light bag on pages 63–68.

Party Time

This is where you have no choice but to remain flexible. When your children are out of the home and with their friends, they are going to be eating whatever's on the go, which is probably not the healthiest food in the world. Don't be overly critical—you only risk making forbidden foods even more desirable. Just keep the 75 Percent Solution in mind. If they eat green-light at home, they can top up on red-light treats from time to time. They know what's good for them and what isn't. Let them make their own decisions. You're the role model, not the rule enforcer!

Is Your Child Overweight?

While the increase in overweight and obesity statistics among adults has been dramatic, it's even more alarming in the case of children. As I said at the beginning of the chapter, 37 percent of Canadian children aged two to eleven are overweight, and 18 percent are technically obese. Obesity has tripled over the past two decades, with Newfoundland topping the Canadian scales.

This is not the place, however, to go into the complex reasons behind the epidemic of childhood obesity. We can blame sedentary habits, video games, and the lack of organized sports activities in school. We can point the finger at TV, and certainly the fast food and advertising industries have a lot to answer for. We eat more and move less. Recent research suggests that only 3 percent of adults adhere to the top four behaviours that characterize healthy lifestyle: maintaining a healthy weight, engaging in regular physical activity, eating more than five servings of fruits and vegetables daily, and not smoking.

Any of those sound familiar to you? Perhaps the best way to address the issue of weight control in your child is to address it in your own life first. However, before you lower the boom, make sure your child really is overweight by discussing the issue with your doctor or pediatrician. I have included some BMI charts in appendix IV that will help you identify whether weight is a problem for your child. But you should then confirm your result with your medical adviser.

All right. Let's say your child is definitely overweight.

The next step is to identify why. Obesity is like a stool with three legs: genetics, diet and exercise. Obviously, we can't do anything about your child's genes, but as parents, we can have a huge impact on the other two factors. There *are* steps you can take to help your child lose weight and feel better. As a parent you must:

1. Recognize there is a problem, i.e., that your child is overweight.
2. Recognize that being obese is emotionally and socially hard on your child.
3. Recognize that this is going to affect the long-term health of your child.
4. Recognize that being fat is going to make a difference to your child's performance in school.
5. Recognize that it is your responsibility to help your child.
6. Recognize that what you say is not as important as what you do.
7. Recognize that food cannot become a battleground, because you will lose.
8. Recognize that you need to plan and work *with* your child, not against him or her. You're on the same team.
9. Recognize that your child is going to need your love, support and optimism to make positive changes.

Diet

There's nothing complicated about the formula for getting fat: if you consume more calories than you expend, you will gain weight. If your child is overweight, he is eating more calories than he burns. Simple. What is more complex is why this should be the case.

When children overeat on a steady basis, there could be many possible contributing factors. Are they unhappy? Bored? Are there family tensions around food, such as arguments and broken rules? Are you a mother whose inability to lose weight causes you to come down hard on other family members who overeat? Or perhaps your child resorts to overeating because of conflict in the marriage that gets acted out at the dinner table. No wonder kids in unhappy households turn to food for comfort.

Eating high-G.I. foods in particular provides a sugar rush and a temporary lift, and eases the emotional pain. But this soon evaporates, as insulin kicks in and blood sugar levels drop, and soon your "comfort eater" is looking for his next sugar fix.

One thing you can do for your overweight child is not to single him out. A child with a weight problem is already under intense social pressure from peers and society in general. As a result, he tends to have low self-esteem, poor self-image and frequently suffers from depression, too. The last thing he needs is for you to be on his case.

The answer is to make weight loss a family affair. Introduce everyone, thin or fat, to eating the green-light way. Make it a project you all share and part of a larger focus on family outings or activities, so it's not just about food. If the new diet comes with more weekends spent together enjoying active fun, it will feel like a change for the better, instead of a good-for-you regime.

Try to avoid even using the word "diet," because this word immediately sets children up for success or failure. Just let them know that you are going to pay more attention to how the whole family eats.

The G.I. Diet can accommodate different goals, because family members who are overweight can follow Phase I, while those who don't have to lose weight can expand their food choices and portions by following Phase II, i.e., adding yellow-light foods to their menus.

If both parents are overweight, there is an 80 percent risk that their children will be overweight. This in turn means that if your children need the G.I. Diet, chances are you or your spouse do, too. At least this makes it easier for everyone to get with the program.

The G.I. Diet, with its emphasis on the good carbs found in fruits, vegetables, legumes and whole grains; on proteins low in saturated fat, such as turkey, chicken, seafood, lean cuts of meat and low-fat dairy; and on limiting unhealthy saturated fats while promoting polyunsaturated and monounsaturated fats, such as those found in nuts and vegetable oils, provides everything your family needs. With children, you should increase the amount of good fats in their diet, since these are essential for nourishing growth. You can do this by including 100% peanut butter in their diet. Although it's a yellow-light food for adults because of its high caloric content, it is a low-G.I. food and an excellent source of protein and good fat. But avoid regular and "light" versions, as some of the peanut content has been replaced with cheaper, unhealthy ingredients, including sugar and starch fillers. All-peanut versions of peanut butter are readily available in supermarkets and health food stores. You need to stir it on opening to keep the oil from separating, but it is the healthiest version.

Exercise

This is the third leg of the stool. To control weight, you need to make sure that the amount of calories consumed is not greater than the energy expended. So to tackle a weight problem, you need to focus on a diet that delivers sound nutrition without excess calories, and you need to be active enough to burn off what you eat. We've lost track of this simple equation. Food is all too ubiquitous, and active fun has a lot of competition from sedentary pleasures like watching TV or playing video games. The multichannel universe has offered children more reasons for not getting off the couch. Nowadays, the importance of the Internet to schoolwork and the popularity of on-line chatting mean that children and teenagers spend a huge amount of their time moving nothing but their fingers over a keyboard.

Research shows that children who spend more than five hours a day in front of the TV are nearly five times more likely to become overweight than those who watch two hours or less. TV watching not only means less activity; it means more eating, in the form of snacks. TV ads aimed at kids don't help either. You don't see many ads selling apples to children.

In many ways, exercise should be "sold" in the same way you encourage good nutrition. In other words, it's up to you to get off the couch first and be the role model. It won't do to have the remote in your hand as you tell your kids to go play outside for a change. The best way to get them out there, with younger children at least, is to head off to the nearest park or playground together. Join in on the kids' games. Play baseball with them. Run around the bases. Play tennis with them. Teach the dog to catch a Frisbee.

Bicycling is another activity that kids and adults can enjoy together. If your kids are under ten, stick to bike paths rather than city streets. If you have kids too young to manoeuvre their own bikes, there's a wide variety of bike buggies available, allowing you to pedal while toddlers get a free and breezy ride. Starting out on the bike paths is also a good way to teach kids bike safety rules before they hit the streets. And bicycling offers you and your family a chance to visit and explore parks and communities outside your neighbourhood. The important thing is to pick a bike frame that fits you, and to adjust the seat so that your leg is extended when the pedal is down. The wrong seat height or too small a bike can put a lot of pressure on the knees.

Are you up for inline skating? If your teenager is into this, you can always accompany him or her on your bike and head for the nearest bike path. As for skateboarding, you should probably leave that to the fifteen-year-old kids, although grown-ups can often learn to snowboard (if they don't mind falling many, many times in the process). If your kids are keen on snowboarding, go with them to the hills and cross-country ski while they hit the slopes. Take your cues from your children and their enthusiasms, then find a way to participate if you can. If your teenage son has learned to kayak at a summer camp, you could plan to rent kayaks and make it a weekend family camping trip. It's easier to try to accommodate to their passions rather than ask them to adopt yours. And you might learn something!

Swimming is wonderful exercise, good for both toning muscles and aerobic conditioning. Sign your kids up for swim classes, and sign yourself up for aquabics classes, which feature gentle exercises done in a shallow pool. Some gyms even schedule adult classes in one pool at the same time as kids' classes in a training pool. Of course, nothing compares with swimming outside, in a lake or pool. If you're lucky enough to have access to a summer cottage, swimming can be something you enjoy all summer long.

Kids just need a nudge to be active. It's what their bodies crave. You'll find you're all in a better mood at the end of a physical day. And you might realize just how dampening TV can be to time spent together as a family. No one is asking you to eliminate TV altogether; just put limits on it. When you get home from a major expedition on bikes, you can make the rental of a video or DVD a special event, rather than let TV be your regular default position.

Sports

If you're lucky enough to have an active child involved in aerobic sports, then being overweight should be less of a problem. However, this is one of the few areas where extra dietary care is needed. Demanding sports like long-distance running, soccer and hockey involve a high expenditure of energy over a long period, and can quickly exhaust the glycogen reserves (the short-term medium for readily available glucose, which feeds the muscles). These reserves should be replenished by a sugar-sweetened drink with electrolytes, such as Gatorade, immediately following the activity. Basically, the sport puts you in "glucose debt," and a sweetened drink helps put you back on track. This is one of the very few times when sugar consumption is a good idea!

TO SUM UP

- Be a role model for your kids. Make your food choices, serving sizes, dining behaviour and exercise habits the kind you want your children to imitate.
- Be responsible and share responsibility. You are responsible for providing meals, and for when and where they are served. Your children are responsible for what and how much they eat. If you try to control everything they eat, food will become a battleground, where everyone loses.
- Make it a family affair. Don't single out the child who needs to lose the weight. This is not a diet. It's a healthy, nutritious way of eating for the whole family, with the welcome side effect of weight loss for those who aim at that.

CHAPTER TEN

When I'm Sixty-Four (or More)

The G.I. Diet and Seniors

If you have an elderly family member living with you, can he or she follow the G.I. Diet, too? Should you recommend it to your seventy-eight-year-old father, who lives alone and doesn't like to cook? What are the special nutritional needs of seniors, and how does being overweight differ in its health impact on the elderly? These are all subjects that aren't often addressed by diet books. But if you are over sixty-five and concerned about your weight, or if you are a caregiver for someone in this stage of life, then these are important questions.

The short answer is yes, the G.I. Diet is both healthy and safe for the elderly. While the low-carb, high-fat regimes may strain the heart health of seniors, and extremely low-fat diets may rob them of the nutrients they require to maintain muscle mass and energy, the G.I. Diet provides a balance that works well for the changing metabolism and nutritional demands of age.

We are only beginning to learn (and research) how the elderly may differ in the way their bodies process fats and protein. But until we know more, the G.I. Diet guarantees a varied range of nutritious food groups and is not confusing to master or follow. The first consideration, as with other age groups, is the risk that obesity poses for those over sixty-five.

One American study has indicated that the number of obese adults over sixty will rise from 14.6 million in 2000 to 20.9 million in 2010—a 43 percent increase. We can anticipate a similar increase in Canada. And the lifetime medical costs for obese men and women will be 42 to 56 percent higher than for people of normal weight.

But the effect of obesity on the personal health of seniors is more costly. Obesity is associated with a greater risk of diabetes, cardiovascular disease, hypertension, stroke, osteoarthritis and some cancers. Furthermore, being overweight restricts the pleasures of physical activity and mobility, and, oddly enough, being overweight doesn't necessarily guarantee sound nutrition either. One study of 2,000 older patients by the Geisinger Medical Center in Danville, Pennsylvania, found that over three hundred of them were obese, with a BMI of 30 or higher. But what was surprising about their nutritional findings was that many overweight and obese older women, especially those living alone, had poor diet quality and didn't get enough fibre, folate, magnesium, iron or zinc, while consuming too much saturated fat. So being fat can coexist with being undernourished.

But enough of the bad news. There *is* an upside to getting old. If you make it past seventy-five, you actually become less of a candidate for obesity. Among those over seventy-five, only 14 percent are obese and 32 percent are overweight. That's lower than the average for those younger!

And the chances of making it to seventy-five have improved, too. A hundred years ago, the average life expectancy was forty-nine years. For women today, it is approaching eighty, and for men the mid-seventies. Most of you reading this chapter will make it (in one shape or another!) to eighty-five. Whether you feel well and enjoy life at that age will have much to do with your ability to maintain a healthy weight.

As Dr. Edward L. Schneider, dean of the school of gerontology at the University of South Carolina, explores in his excellent book, *AgeLess*, the greatest fear around aging is not death but disability. At eighty-five, half of us will need outside help for bathing, dressing, walking, meal preparation and even going to the toilet. This is not a happy prospect. What can we do to help prevent this fate? Ill health isn't something we can totally eliminate, but addressing the issue of nutrition in old age, and preventing obesity, can definitely make a difference in how we navigate our senior years. Obesity sets up a domino effect: if you're too heavy to exercise, your bone strength suffers, resulting in a higher risk of fractures if you fall. Limited activity also affects mood and contributes to another scourge of old age: depression. Keeping the pounds off is one of the most effective ways to arm yourself against the slings and arrows of old age.

So we know that being overweight is hard on your body. But new research has also found a direct link between a high BMI and the risk of developing dementia. In a recent issue of *Archives of Internal Medicine,* Swedish researchers found that for subjects with a BMI of 30 or higher, the risk of developing dementia was two and half times greater. If the goal of looking better no longer motivates you at seventy, perhaps the hope of thinking better will!

But—and this is the unfair part about aging—as you get older it only gets harder to shed extra weight. It's not your willpower crumbling; your metabolism and body requirements are shifting. This is a different stage of life, with its own biochemical signature. So let's take a look at why we put on weight as we age.

You may be eating the same and exercising the way you always have (or haven't), and yet after forty, the tape measure turns treacherous. The size ten pants go to the back of the closet, and the skirt that used to flatter your hips now doesn't. If you once enjoyed the classic proportion of 38–28–38, it's more likely to go south and settle on your hips: 38–30–41 is more like it in middle age. (I suppose that's why they call it middle age: that's where all the pounds go!)

Dear Rick,

I started on the G.I. Diet after seeing the success my daughter had on it. I bought the book and immediately started to lose weight regularly at 2 pounds a week. I am now sixty-five years old, 5 feet 7 inches tall and have lost over 35 pounds and gone down three dress sizes. At the same time, I have never eaten so well. This isn't like a diet, it just seems to be a healthier way of eating. I am determined to never let myself get fat again as I feel so much better. Before I lost the weight I had constant indigestion and didn't sleep well. Losing weight has, for me, been a great morale booster—I feel so much better about myself.

Pat

So the percentage of body fat goes up and the proportion of lean muscle tissue goes down. In terms of muscle, we peak in our twenties. From then on, it's downhill, as we lose about 2 percent of our muscle mass with every decade. In middle age, this loss quickly accelerates. For a forty-year-old woman or a sixty-year-old man, the loss of muscle increases by 6 to 8 percent per decade. Since muscle burns more calories than fat, you're also losing that benefit as well. You're burning up fewer calories, just when you might be tempted to take in more.

Your energy may not be the same either. You might find you have to do more of the less strenuous forms of activity rather than the high-energy activities you did when you were young. The irony is that as we age, it's going to take more time and effort to simply maintain our shape, let alone improve it. But don't worry about a few extra pounds; they might come in handy during a period of illness or as a cushion against falls and fractures.

If we recalibrate the way we eat and how much to reflect the changing metabolism of aging, it's possible to control our weight and to stay active as well, which is the key to good health and happiness as we age. We tend to become less active the older we get. For men, active sports like hockey or soccer are replaced by more leisurely ones like golf. Retirement also eliminates the routine activities of the working day. Women who did the physical work of maintaining a household and caring for children may find themselves idling in an empty nest. No more multiple trips up and down the stairs with laundry or chasing after toddlers in the park. Our metabolism slows just as our activities begin to slow down as well. (Some studies have found that the metabolic rate can decline as much as 30 percent over a lifetime.)

So at the age of seventy, your body has less muscle, and therefore requires fewer calories. It may use dietary protein less efficiently, and you might also have some digestive issues—heartburn, constipation, irritable bowel syndrome—that discourage you from eating a proper diet. Poor dental health can dampen the appetite, as can depression and loneliness. Older widowed people may not feel motivated to cook for themselves, and with age, our sense of taste and smell grow less acute. All of these factors can interfere with eating healthily.

Before we explore how the G.I. Diet can help seniors, let's discuss the appropriate BMI for someone over sixty. As with children, there are mitigating factors involved. Some extra body fat, as I mentioned earlier, may help prevent hip fractures in case of a fall, and tide you over during a period of illness. So when you set your BMI target, you may want to aim for the higher side of normal. While the average BMI for most people is 22, you might want to raise yours to 24 or 25. This will give you an extra ten pounds or so. There is now some evidence that people with a slightly higher BMI may live longer. In any case, don't berate yourself if you can't maintain that perfect BMI of 22. It might be the wisdom of age at work in your body.

Nutritional Needs

Older people need to pay particular attention to how much vitamin D, calcium and vitamin B12 their diet delivers. The body needs more calcium as it ages, to keep the bones strong and to reduce the risk of osteoporosis. Calcium may also help maintain healthy blood pressure and play a role in preventing colon cancer. Seniors should get about 1,200 milligrams of calcium a day, and women should get 1,500 milligrams, the equivalent of five glasses of milk. You can also get calcium by eating almonds, canned salmon (with the bones), calcium-enriched soy milk or orange juice, and leafy green vegetables such as kale, spinach and Swiss chard.

But to make calcium available to the bones, you need vitamin D, which is obtained through exposure to sunlight. Canadians who spend the winters indoors may not get enough sunlight to acquire the recommended amount of 800 IU a day. Sunscreens also reduce the effect by cutting down the essential UV rays. And, as we age, the skin's ability to convert sunlight into vitamin D declines. It might take ten times the exposure to sun for seniors to achieve the same vitamin D levels they had in their youth. (Perhaps this is why seniors naturally gravitate to the sunshine states!) Our need for this vitamin doubles after age fifty, and triples after age seventy. Vitamin D is also important for the prevention of cancer, including breast and colon.

Fortunately, the dairy industry adds vitamin D to all its products. But even on the G.I. Diet, which includes low-fat dairy and deep-sea fish, another good source, you probably won't get enough vitamin D. The simplest solution, then, is to take a daily multivitamin as insurance.

To illustrate the importance of this vitamin, consider an American study of seniors' diets, conducted at Tufts University. The group was in the lower half of the normal range of vitamin D levels. Half of them then received a vitamin D supplement, while half took a placebo. The group given vitamin D suffered half as many injuries from falls. This is significant, since falls are the most common form of injury after the age of sixty-five and are a leading cause of death and disability. Women in particular are vulnerable to hip fractures, and one in five will die as a direct result. So for postmenopausal women, a calcium supplement, in combination with vitamin D, is a good idea.

The other elusive element in old age is vitamin B12, which is essential for heart health and stroke prevention. About a third of older people lack the stomach acid to properly absorb this vitamin from their diet alone, so a separate vitamin B supplement is recommended (the amount in a multivitamin is not enough). Iron deficiency causes 15 to 30 percent of anemia in seniors, but another 10 percent is caused by B12 deficiency.

Digestion also changes as we get older, because we produce fewer digestive enzymes. Our bodies normally produce twenty-two different digestive enzymes, and the foods we eat contain many more. Each enzyme acts on a specific type of food. Protease, for example, helps break down proteins; amylase helps us digest carbohydrates; lipase goes to work on fats, and cellulase, found in plants, helps us digest fibre. This is why products such as Lactaid (lactase) help people who have a problem digesting dairy products and why Beano (cellulase) helps prevent gas in people who don't process fibre well. When we produce fewer digestive enzymes, symptoms such as bloating, indigestion, heartburn and gas become more familiar. We start popping more Rolaids and Tums, and thinking twice before eating spicy foods.

There's no simple answer to this decrease in enzyme

production as we age. Taking multiple digestive enzymes won't help since they are mainly destroyed by acids in the stomach. Eating slowly in a relaxed situation and chewing thoroughly are probably your best aid to digestion (a glass of red wine might also help).

Since older adults also have a decreased sensation of thirst, it pays to make a habit of taking lots of fluids— water, milk, tea or clear soup. Dehydration can lead to constipation, another nuisance that comes with age.

With these supplements and nutritional advice in mind, then, following the G.I. Diet is an excellent way for seniors to stay on track, both in terms of weight management and optimum health.

Staying Active

Let's be quite clear about this: if you want to maintain a healthy weight, live longer and prevent disability and dependence in your old age, exercise is not an option, it's a must. But it doesn't have to mean running marathons, lifting dumbbells or enduring disco-driven aerobics classes. There are all kinds of pleasant, low-key ways to include physical activity in your life.

A few years ago, the advice regarding exercise was "no pain, no gain." You had to sweat, sprint, get your heart rate up and push your limit. Recent evidence, however, suggests that any activity is better than none, and that thirty minutes of brisk walking a day can be just as beneficial as

Dear Rick,

I am a seventy-year-old man and have been on various diets and weight control programs for most of my life. Until the G.I. Diet, each one had limited effect and failed in one way or another. I have now been on the G.I. Diet for four months, and have lost approximately 15 kilograms in six months. Never have I felt hungry or deprived. On the contrary, I think I eat more now than before! I also have reduced my waist measurement by 4 inches and weigh less than I did when I joined the RCAF at age eighteen! As well, my blood sugar levels are controlled without medication, and my blood pressure is down as well as cholesterol. Bonus! The renewed energy and feeling of well-being are amazing. I recommend this diet to everyone, even if weight loss is not the prime goal. I will be on this program for the rest of my life.

Thank you!

Gordon

more intense workouts. The only problem with exercise for older adults is that the benefits tend to evaporate rather quickly, so you have to be active on a regular basis. In your youth, you could get away with a lapse in activity and the muscles might not even notice. At the age of seventy, however, a lazy week will reverse all the hard work you've done maintaining muscle tone. And more important than having shapely calves, you want to sustain an independent lifestyle as long as you can. Other than diet, the single best thing you can do to ensure this is to get off the couch. The risk of nearly all the "old-age" diseases—cancer, heart, stroke, diabetes, dementia—are significantly reduced by exercise. Yes, a glass of wine with dinner and a good laugh at a sitcom on TV are good for your health too, but only in combination with daily activity. The secret is to find an exercise you enjoy doing. There are three areas of exercise that complement one another. **Note: You should talk to your doctor before embarking on an exercise program.**

1. Aerobic/Cardio

Aerobic exercise—walking up a flight of stairs is one example—works your heart, lungs and muscles all at once. At the gym, you can get an aerobic workout by swimming or using the treadmill, cross-trainer or stair climber machine. Some machines will even tell you, by combining your weight and age, what your target heart rate should be and when the aerobic benefits kick in. You don't want to exercise too strenuously.

You can also work on a stationary bicycle at home. But many seniors are already socially isolated, so sometimes joining a gym offers not only exercise but a sense of community as well. The YMCA has a number of programs designed especially for older adults, including aquabics, where gentle exercises are done in a heated pool. The Y also offers a degree of subsidy for those who can't afford the fees. Many gyms and clubs have all-female facilities, which are popular with older women who don't want to work out in a sea of fit young athletes.

If you're not the gym type, you can get your aerobic exercise simply by making a habit of walking briskly—as if you were late for an appointment—every day for thirty minutes. If the weather is nasty, try "mall aerobics": drive to the nearest mall and walk from one end to the other and back. For the truly enterprising, jogging, biking and cross-country skiing are endurance sports that can be enjoyed into old age. Jackrabbit Johannsen, the famous Norwegian-Canadian cross-country skier, participated in ski marathons well into his eighties and nineties (and lived to be 111!)

2. Strength Training

Lifting weights helps you maintain strong bones and keeps your muscles toned. In a gym, ask the staff to make sure you are using the strength-training equipment properly. Some people assume that pushing heavier weights will get faster results, but you set yourself up for injuries if you do this. The key to strength training is to start small, using lots of repetitions with low weights. Increase the number of repetitions rather than adding more weights.

At home, use a set of two-, three- and five-pound weights. A yoga mat helps with balance and traction. Thera-Bands—stretchy rubber sashes that you use during exercise to create resistance—are good for gentle strength training, too.

The exercise system known as Pilates is also excellent for older people, because it lets you go at your own speed. Developed by dancers for strengthening the body and dealing with injuries, this technique is as demanding or as gentle as your body requires. It focuses on increasing your core strength, the abdominal and back muscles in particular. It's a wonderful way to prevent or diminish lower back pain, and it has postural benefits as well.

3. Stretching/Flexibility

Stretching is good for muscles, tendons, ligaments and joints. As well, it helps in the general aches and pains department, making stair climbing and housework easier. Staying flexible also develops your balance and minimizes potential injuries from falls.

Why do falls happen? Sometimes, it's as simple as not lifting the front of your foot high enough as you take a step. This can happen when your calf muscles lose flexibility, which is particularly the case for women after a lifetime of wearing high heels. You begin to shuffle rather than lift the foot, and this makes it easier for you to catch your toe and fall.

I often find helpful suggestions for exercise, diet and food shopping in an excellent publication called *Nutrition Action* (you can find details at www.cspinet.org). The newsletter also provides detailed and very useful product information; I recommend it highly. In the December 2002 issue, for instance, one contributor suggested that seniors who neglect stretching often become round-shouldered. Osteoporosis is the likely culprit with curved spines, but regular stretching can help combat this tendency. Stretching alone can result in a 100 percent increase in flexibility in just one week!

Any gym will offer advice on simple stretching exercises, but one of the best ways to stay supple is to join a yoga class. One weekly yoga class can do wonders, not only for lower back pain but also for posture, stress and mood. The emphasis on deep, regular breathing is also nourishing to the muscles and relaxing. Once you learn the ropes in class, yoga exercises are also easy to do at home. You're never too old to enjoy the benefits of this ancient practice.

TO SUM UP

- The G.I. Diet will help seniors lose weight and keep it off.
- If you improve your health, you'll reduce your risk of falling prey to today's major diseases and disabilities.
- Take a multivitamin to address possible calcium and vitamin D deficiencies. A vitamin B supplement is also recommended.
- Incorporate some aerobic exercise, strength training and stretching into your routine. Remember, use it or lose it!

CHAPTER ELEVEN

How Your Family G.I. Diet Can Fight Disease

Foods are fuel and a source of pleasure, too. But food can also have a biochemical effect on us that's as powerful as any drug. Everything we eat affects our health, well-being and emotional state, and this happens four or five times a day. Most of the time, we're looking for the pleasure angle rather than biochemistry. Imagine if we went to the medicine cabinet and chose our drugs the same way! The right foods can help you lose and maintain your weight, protect your health, extend your lifespan, give you more energy and make you feel good and sleep better. Couple that with exercise and you are doing all you can to keep healthy, fit and alert. The rest is a matter of genes and luck.

Let's take a look at how diet acts as a critical factor in preventing some familiar diseases.

Heart Disease and Stroke

These are the two biggies. Heart disease and stroke account for 40 percent of all deaths in North America. Nearly half of those who suffer heart attacks are under the age of sixty-five. And the simple fact is that many of those heart attacks could have been prevented by diet.

The more overweight you are, the more likely it is you will suffer a heart attack or stroke. The key factors linking these two diseases to diet are cholesterol and hypertension (high blood pressure). I won't go into the detailed science here, but everyone should understand a little bit about the role and significance of cholesterol and hypertension.

One of the harbingers of both heart attack and stroke is high blood pressure, or hypertension. Think of the arterial system as a garden hose where the force of the water is too great. With hypertension, there is too much stress on the arterial system, which causes it to age and deteriorate too rapidly. This eventually leads to arterial damage, blood clots and a heart attack or stroke. In simple terms, a blockage in an artery to the heart triggers a heart attack (not enough blood and oxygen reach the heart), and a blockage in an artery going to or in the brain will cause a stroke.

Why are we talking about medical matters in a diet book? Because excess weight has a major bearing on blood pressure, which in turn can trigger these life-threatening diseases. A recent study demonstrated that a lower-fat diet, coupled with a sizable increase in fruits and vegetables (eight to ten servings a day), lowered blood pressure.

In other words, the G.I. Diet is the way to lower your blood pressure and reduce your risk of disease.

As for cholesterol, it has a bad reputation, but we need to understand its role more clearly. Cholesterol itself is essential to your body's metabolism, and we can't live without it. But high levels of cholesterol contribute to the plaque that builds up in your arteries, eventually causing blockage.

To make things more complicated, as you probably know there are two forms of cholesterol: HDL (the good kind) and LDL (the bad). The idea is to boost HDL while suppressing LDL. (One way to remember the difference: HDL is "Heart's Delight Level," and LDL is "Leads to Death Level.") And what pushes the LDL levels up into the danger zone? Saturated fat. The kind that turns solid at room temperature—like the stuff you skim off chicken soup and the lovely white lard you bake into a pie crust. This is also what marbles tasty steak and makes bacon sizzle in the pan. Saturated fat is also present in whole milk and hidden in crackers and pretzels.

Polyunsaturated and monounsaturated fats work to lower LDL levels, and also actually boost HDL. So make sure that the right sort of fat is part of what you eat (see page 17).

Diabetes

Diabetes is the kissing cousin of heart disease, in the sense that more people die of heart complications arising from having diabetes than from diabetes alone. And diabetes rates are skyrocketing: they are expected to double in the next ten years.

The most common form of diabetes is called Type 2; it used to be called Adult Onset Diabetes as well, but now so many children are developing diabetes that the name had to be changed. The main causes of the alarming rise in Type 2 diabetes are obesity and lack of exercise. The most dramatic illustration of this link can be seen in the incidence of diabetes among North American's Native population. It affects nearly half of them. Before the Europeans arrived on this continent, Aboriginal peoples lived in a natural state of feast or famine. When food was abundant, whether from plants or animal sources, it was stored as body fat. Then, in lean times, such as winter, the body drew on these fat supplies. As a result of this cycle, they developed a "thrift gene"; those who stored and used their food most efficiently became the best survivors, a clear example of Darwin's survival of the fittest.

But when you take away the need to hunt or harvest food—in other words, being physically active—with a convenient supermarket you can drive to, the result is predictable: more people are going to eat more, move less, become obese and develop diabetes. The fact that we are a culture in love with sugar contributes to this chain of events as well.

Now we know that eating a low-G.I. diet releases sugar more slowly into the bloodstream and helps stabilize blood sugar levels, which, in turn, helps control diabetes. This way of eating has the additional advantage of helping diabetics lose weight, which is significant considering that the most common cause of diabetes in the first place is overweight. But even though the G.I. Diet is helpful for managing diabetes, prevention is far preferable. That's where low-G.I. eating is really valuable.

Cancer

Every year, the evidence mounts for the assertion that weight and diet are critical risk factors for most forms of cancer. Diets high in animal fats (saturated), such as the low-carb, high-protein regimes that have been popular, are directly associated with increased vulnerability to breast, colon and prostate cancers. On the other hand, people who eat more fresh vegetables, fruits and whole grains seem to have a lower risk of developing these cancers. The American Institute for Cancer Research recommends that people eat a predominantly plant-based diet that includes a variety of vegetables, fruits and grains—in other words, the G.I. Diet.

Alzheimer's

Over the past two to three years, there has been a steady flow of research studies linking Alzheimer's and dementia to diet. A diet high in saturated fat can double the risk of getting this dreadful disease. As we mentioned earlier, anyone with a BMI of 30 or higher is two and a half times more likely to develop dementia. (Note: This study was based on data from more than seven thousand men. We don't know the implications for women.) Alcohol, salt and refined carbs were also associated with risk.

On the upside, a diet rich in deep-sea fish (i.e., oily

fish, such as sardines, mackerel and herring) can help prevent Alzheimer's. It seems that the omega-3 oil and vitamin E found in these fish are the helpful agents. Many studies also suggest that the anti-inflammatory effect of antioxidants found in nuts and green vegetables, such as spinach, broccoli and Brussels sprouts, may have a protective effect against Alzheimer's.

Well, you know the bottom line here: the G.I. Diet is low in saturated fat and rich in omega-3 and vitamin E. It's your best line of defence against the loss of your cognitive abilities and memory in advanced age.

Arthritis

Diet again seems to be very helpful in managing arthritis, especially osteoarthritis. Being overweight already puts a strain on joints, especially weight-bearing ones. What if your knees, hips and ankles have to absorb an extra fifty to sixty pounds of impact every time your foot hits the ground? Try lifting a fifty-pound weight and you'll see what your poor body is coping with. Don't make your joints work harder than they have to.

Abdominal Fat

The most alarming medical news about fat, which runs contrary to our popular assumptions, is that it is not a passive accumulator of energy or extra baggage. Rather, it is an active, living part of your body. Once it accumulates enough mass, fat behaves very much like any of the body organs, such as the liver, heart or kidneys, except that it actively undermines your health by pumping out a dangerous combination of free fatty acids and proteins. This causes rapid cell proliferation, which is associated with the growth of malignant cancer tumours. In other words, fat seems to spur the growth of cancer, when those cells are present.

Fat also creates inflammation, which is linked to atherosclerosis (artery thickening), which in turn causes heart disease and stroke. It also increases insulin resistance, which leads to Type 2 diabetes. So a beer belly, or "apple shape," is not just an inert lump of fat. These tissues behave more like a huge tumour, actively undermining health in other parts of your body. Not a pleasant thought.

Prostate Health

Just as a low-fat diet can help protect women from developing breast cancer, a diet low in saturated fat has been shown to offer protection to men from prostate cancer, which is even more pervasive among older men. Eating too much red meat puts men at higher risk of both colon and prostate cancer. A diet low in animal fats and high in fresh fruits and vegetables is a prostate-friendly diet—in other words, the G.I. Diet.

Part III:

Recipes

Breakfast

GRANOLA-TOPPED PEACHES   GREEN-LIGHT

Eating fresh fruit for breakfast gives you a healthy start
to the day. In this dish, peaches are combined with granola and cottage cheese for an additional energy boost.
They can also be served cold.

1/2 cup	large-flake rolled oats
1/4 cup	sliced almonds
1/4 cup	All-Bran or 100% Bran cereal
6	ripe peaches
1 tbsp	soft non-hydrogenated margarine
1	tub (500 g) non-fat cottage cheese
1/4 cup	dried cranberries or raisins
2 tbsp	sugar substitute
2 tsp	grated orange rind

1. In non-stick skillet, toast rolled oats and almonds over
   medium heat, stirring constantly, for about 8 minutes
   or until golden brown. Place in bowl. Add cereal and
   set aside.

2. Meanwhile, cut peaches in half horizontally and remove pit. Melt margarine in large non-stick skillet over medium heat. Place peaches, cut side down, in skillet and cook for about 5 minutes or until starting to soften. Transfer to platter.
3. In bowl, stir together cottage cheese, cranberries, sugar substitute and orange rind. Spoon evenly over peach halves. Sprinkle with granola mixture.

Makes 6 servings.

Canned Peach Option: You can substitute 12 canned large peach halves, drained, for the fresh peaches. Omit the cooking step for the peaches.

Pear Option: Try using 6 ripe Bartlett pears instead of the peaches. Nectarines would also work well.

ORANGE BERRY WAFFLES

This simple recipe freezes well, so be sure to make extra waffles for weekday breakfasts. A couple of slices of back bacon on the side add protein to the meal.

1/3 cup	whole wheat flour
3/4 cup	wheat bran
2 tbsp	sugar substitute
1/4 tsp	cinnamon
Pinch	salt
1 1/4 cups	skim milk
1/3 cup	liquid eggs
1 tsp	vanilla
1/3 cup	liquid egg whites

Orange Berry Compote:

2	oranges, peeled
1 cup	sliced strawberries, fresh or frozen
1 cup	fresh or frozen blueberries
3 tbsp	water
3 tbsp	sugar substitute
2 tbsp	cornstarch

I. **Orange Berry Compote:** Chop oranges and place, along with juice, in saucepan. Add strawberries, blueberries, water, sugar substitute and cornstarch. Bring to boil, stirring occasionally. Cook for about 1 minute or until thickened. Remove from heat.

2. In bowl, whisk together flour, bran, sugar substitute, cinnamon and salt; set aside. In another bowl, whisk together milk, liquid eggs and vanilla; pour over flour mixture and whisk until combined.
3. In another bowl, beat liquid egg whites until stiff peaks form. Fold into batter.
4. Heat waffle iron. Spray lightly with cooking spray and pour in about ½ cup of the batter. Close lid and cook for about 4 minutes or until steam stops and waffle is golden. Repeat with remaining batter. Serve with compote.

Makes 6 to 8 servings.

Storage: Waffles can be wrapped individually and frozen for up to 1 month. Reheat in microwave or, for a crisper waffle, in toaster. Orange Berry Compote can be refrigerated for up to 2 days and reheated over low heat or in the microwave.

MINI BREAKFAST PUFFS

Ideal for those rushed mornings, these muffin-sized puffs are packed with nutrition.

1 tsp	canola oil
¼ cup	diced onion
1	red bell pepper, diced
1 cup	chopped broccoli
½ tsp	dried thyme
¼ tsp	each salt and pepper
¾ cup	crumbled light feta cheese
1 ½ cups	liquid eggs
1 cup	skim milk
¼ cup	wheat bran
¼ cup	whole wheat flour

1. In non-stick skillet, heat oil over medium heat. Cook onion and red pepper for about 5 minutes or until softened. Add broccoli, thyme, salt and pepper; cover and steam for about 3 minutes or until tender-crisp and bright green. Divide mixture among 12 greased muffin tins; set aside.
2. Sprinkle cheese over top of vegetable mixture.
3. In bowl, whisk together liquid eggs, milk, bran and whole wheat flour. Pour evenly over vegetable mixture. Bake in 400° F oven for about 20 minutes or until golden, set and puffed. Let cool slightly before serving.

Makes 12 puffs (6 to 8 servings).

Storage: These muffins can be made up to 3 days ahead and refrigerated; reheat in the microwave for an instant breakfast.

Helpful Hint: For a light lunch have a muffin with a salad.

Cheese Option: Try using light-style Cheddar cheese.

HAM AND ASPARAGUS BREAKFAST BREAD

This bread is a wonderful brunch dish.

1 ½ cups	chopped asparagus
1 ½ cups	whole wheat flour
½ cup	wheat bran
2 tsp	baking powder
¼ tsp	salt
¾ cup	skim milk
½ cup	liquid eggs
¼ cup	soft non-hydrogenated margarine, melted
¾ cup	chopped lean ham or back bacon
2	green onions, chopped

1. In large non-stick skillet, bring ½ cup water to boil; add asparagus. Cover and steam for about 3 minutes or until tender-crisp. Drain and rinse under cold water. Drain well; set aside.

2. In bowl, whisk together flour, bran, baking powder and salt. In another bowl, whisk together milk, liquid eggs and margarine; pour over flour mixture and stir to combine. Stir in cooked asparagus, ham and onions until combined. Pour into greased 9-inch square baking dish and bake in 375° F oven for about 25 minutes or until knife inserted in centre comes out clean.

Makes 9 bars.

EGG AND HAM TORTILLA ROLL-UP   GREEN-LIGHT

These roll-ups are a favourite breakfast and lunch dish, so make stacks of egg pancakes ahead of time and store them in the fridge.

1 tsp	canola oil
1	green onion, chopped
⅓ cup	liquid eggs
Pinch	each salt and pepper
¼ cup	cooked red kidney beans
¼ tsp	dried oregano
1	small whole wheat tortilla
1	slice lean ham or turkey (optional)

1. In small non-stick skillet, heat oil over medium heat. Cook onion for about 1 minute or until softened.
2. Whisk together liquid eggs, salt and pepper. Pour into skillet and stir, using heat-resistant spatula, for about 30 seconds or until beginning to set. Let cook for about 2 minutes or until no longer runny.
3. Meanwhile, in bowl, mash beans and oregano until smooth. Spread over tortilla and top with ham, if using. Slide egg pancake onto ham and roll up.

Makes 1 serving.

VEGETABLE FRITTATA

Frittatas are a great way to get your family to eat their veggies. Use whatever vegetables you have in the fridge to create this nutritious breakfast or lunch dish.

2 tsp	extra-virgin olive oil
1	onion, chopped
2	cloves garlic, minced
1	yellow bell pepper, chopped
1 ½ cups	sliced mushrooms
1 tsp	Italian herb seasoning
Pinch	hot pepper flakes
1 cup	fresh or frozen peas
1 ¼ cups	liquid eggs
¼ tsp	each salt and pepper

1. In non-stick skillet, heat oil over medium heat. Cook onion, garlic, yellow pepper, mushrooms, Italian herb seasoning and hot pepper flakes for about 8 minutes or until liquid evaporates from mushrooms. Add peas and cook for 2 minutes, stirring constantly.
2. In bowl, whisk together liquid eggs, salt and pepper. Pour into skillet, stirring well to combine vegetables and egg mixture. Cook for about 5 minutes, lifting edges to allow uncooked eggs to run underneath, until top is not runny and bottom is golden.
3. Place plate large enough to cover skillet over top and invert pan to remove frittata. Slide frittata back into

skillet and cook for about 5 minutes or until golden and knife inserted in centre comes out clean.

Makes 4 to 6 servings.

Helpful Hint: You can serve wedges of frittata open-faced on whole wheat bread or enjoy with a salad.

Soups

BEEF AND KALE SOUP

GREEN-LIGHT

Kale is a great source of vitamin C and folate. Combine it with beef to make a hearty soup for cold winter days. The brave can add a dash of hot pepper sauce to their servings.

1 tsp	canola oil
1	onion, thinly sliced
2	cloves garlic, minced
1/2 tsp	ground cumin
1/2 tsp	ground coriander
4 cups	beef stock (low-fat, low-sodium)
2 cups	lightly packed finely shredded kale
1	top sirloin grilling steak (about 8 oz)
1	can (540 mL) red kidney beans, drained and rinsed
Pinch	each salt and pepper

1. In stockpot, heat oil over medium heat. Cook onion, garlic, cumin and coriander for about 8 minutes or until softened and beginning to turn golden. Add stock and bring to boil. Add kale and cook, stirring occasionally, for 5 minutes.
2. Meanwhile, trim any fat from steak and discard. Slice steak into thin strips and cut strips in half crosswise. Add to soup along with beans, salt and pepper. Cook, stirring occasionally, for about 10 minutes or until kale is tender and steak is slightly pink inside.

Makes 3 to 4 servings.

Chicken Option: You can substitute 2 boneless skinless chicken breasts, thinly sliced, for the beef; cook until no longer pink inside.

Spinach Option: Use spinach or Swiss chard instead of kale.

Bean Option: Substitute white kidney beans, lentils or black beans for the red kidney beans.

CHICKEN VEGETABLE NOODLE SOUP   GREEN-LIGHT

This soup is the ultimate in comfort food for adults and kids alike. For variety, try it with turkey instead of the chicken.

1 tbsp	canola oil
1	leek, white and light green part only, thinly sliced
2	stalks celery, chopped
1	carrot, chopped
4	cloves garlic, minced
8 oz	mushrooms, sliced
1 tbsp	chopped fresh thyme (or 1 tsp dried)
1/2 tsp	pepper
1/4 tsp	salt
6 cups	chicken stock (low-fat, low-sodium)
3	boneless skinless chicken breasts, diced
1/3 cup	orzo pasta
2 cups	lightly packed shredded spinach
1	can (540 mL) red kidney beans, drained and rinsed

1. In stockpot, heat oil over medium heat. Cook leek for about 5 minutes or until beginning to soften. Add celery, carrot, garlic, mushrooms, thyme, pepper and salt. Cook, stirring, for about 8 minutes or until liquid evaporates from mushrooms and they start to turn golden.

2. Add chicken stock and bring to boil. Add chicken and orzo and cook, stirring occasionally, for about 10 minutes or until chicken is no longer pink inside and pasta is al dente. Add spinach and beans and cook until spinach is wilted and beans are hot.

Makes 6 to 8 servings.

Vegetarian Option: To make this soup vegetarian, substitute vegetable stock for the chicken stock and use 2 cups of diced firm tofu instead of the chicken.

HEARTY LENTIL TOMATO SOUP `GREEN-LIGHT`

This isn't your average thin, watery tomato soup. It's packed with vegetables and is rich in flavour. Fill a thermos for lunch at work or school. For an added kick, sprinkle soup with hot pepper flakes before serving.

2 tsp	canola oil
1	large onion, finely chopped
3	cloves garlic, minced
1	carrot, diced
1	stalk celery, diced
1 tsp	Italian herb seasoning
1 cup	dried green lentils
2 tbsp	tomato paste
6 cups	vegetable stock (low-fat, low-sodium)
1	can (796 mL) diced tomatoes
1 cup	diced firm tofu
1 cup	fresh or frozen peas
¼ tsp	each salt and pepper

1. In stockpot, heat oil over medium heat. Cook onion, garlic, carrot, celery and Italian herb seasoning for about 8 minutes or until softened. Add lentils and tomato paste and cook, stirring, for 2 minutes. Add stock and diced tomatoes and bring to boil. Cover and reduce heat; boil gently for about 1 hour or until lentils are tender.

2. Add tofu, peas, salt and pepper and cook for about 5 minutes or until peas are tender.

    Makes 4 to 6 servings.

Storage: You can freeze this soup for up to 1 month. Thaw in refrigerator and reheat in saucepan or microwave.

Salads

VILLAGE SALAD

GREEN-LIGHT

This is a variation on a classic Greek salad. The addition of beans and hearty greens adds much needed protein and fibre.

4 cups	shredded romaine or escarole lettuce
4	tomatoes, cut in thin wedges
1	green bell pepper, thinly sliced
1	can (540 mL) white kidney beans, drained and rinsed
3/4 cup	diced light feta cheese
Half	cucumber, thinly sliced
1/3 cup	chopped, pitted kalamata olives
2 tbsp	lemon juice
1 tbsp	extra-virgin olive oil
1	clove garlic, minced
1/4 tsp	each salt and pepper
2 tbsp	each chopped fresh oregano and flat-leaf parsley
1 tbsp	chopped fresh mint

1. In large shallow bowl, combine lettuce, tomatoes, green pepper and kidney beans. Top with feta, cucumber and olives.
2. In small bowl, whisk together lemon juice, oil, garlic, salt and pepper. Pour over salad and toss to coat. Add oregano, parsley and mint and toss to combine well.

Makes 4 to 6 servings.

Tuna Option: For more flavour, add 2 cans (120 g each) chunk tuna packed in water, drained.

CHICKPEA AND CHICKEN SALAD   GREEN-LIGHT

Chickpeas and chicken make a great combination. This salad can also be served in half a whole wheat pita with lettuce and tomato slices.

2 tsp	canola oil
¼ cup	chopped fresh flat-leaf parsley
½ tsp	ground cumin
½ tsp	each salt and pepper
2	boneless skinless chicken breasts
1	can (540 mL) chickpeas, drained and rinsed
½ cup	chopped celery
½ cup	each chopped red and green bell pepper
2	green onions, chopped
2 cups	shredded romaine or leaf lettuce
¼ cup	non-fat mayonnaise
3 tbsp	plain non-fat yogurt
¼ tsp	grated lemon rind
1 tbsp	lemon juice
2 tsp	sugar substitute
2 tsp	chili powder
1	small clove garlic, minced

1. In bowl, combine oil, 2 tbsp of the parsley, cumin and half each of the salt and pepper. Add chicken and toss to coat evenly. Place breasts on greased grill over medium-high heat and cook for about 10 minutes or until no longer pink inside. Transfer to plate and set aside.

2. In large bowl, combine chickpeas, celery, red and green peppers, green onions and lettuce. In small bowl, whisk together mayonnaise, yogurt, lemon rind and juice, sugar substitute, chili powder and garlic. Add remaining parsley, salt and pepper. Pour over chickpea mixture and stir to combine.

3. Chop chicken into bite-sized pieces and add to salad. Toss to combine.

Makes 4 servings.

Helpful Hint: You can use leftover chicken for the chicken breasts. You will need 1 ½ cups, chopped.

Turkey Option: Substitute turkey for the chicken.

Tofu Option: Replace the chicken with 1 ½ cups chopped extra-firm tofu (either flavoured or plain).

Cucumber Option: If you don't want to use red or green peppers, substitute 1 cup chopped cucumber.

FOUR-BEAN SALAD

GREEN-LIGHT

Packed with fibre, this classic salad is perfect for lunch or a snack. Make extra to refrigerate for another day.

8 oz	green beans, trimmed
8 oz	yellow beans, trimmed
1	can (540 mL) red kidney beans, drained and rinsed
1	can (540 mL) chickpeas, drained and rinsed
1/2 cup	chopped celery
1/2 cup	diced red onion
1/3 cup	red wine vinegar
2 tbsp	extra-virgin olive oil
2	cloves garlic, minced
1 tbsp	Dijon mustard
1 tsp	celery seed
1/4 tsp	each salt and pepper
1/4 cup	chopped fresh flat-leaf parsley
1/4 cup	chopped fresh mint or basil
2 cups	shredded romaine lettuce
2 cups	baby spinach leaves

1. Cut green and yellow beans into 1-inch pieces. In saucepan of boiling salted water, cook beans for about 7 minutes or until tender-crisp. Drain and rinse under cold water until cool. Drain well. Place in large bowl. Add red kidney beans, chickpeas, celery and onion to bowl.

2. In small bowl, whisk together vinegar, oil, garlic, mustard, celery seed, salt and pepper. Pour over bean mixture. Add parsley and basil. Toss to coat evenly.

3. Combine romaine and spinach and divide among 4 plates. Spoon bean mixture over lettuce mixture to serve.

Makes 4 to 6 servings.

Tofu Option: Omit 1 can of beans and add 1 ½ cups diced extra-firm tofu to the salad.

WHEAT BERRY APPLE CRANBERRY SALAD

Wheat berries are whole wheat kernels and are high in fibre. When mixed with apples and tart cranberries, the result is a definite winner.

1 cup	wheat berries
2	Granny Smith apples, cored and diced
2 cups	lightly packed baby spinach
1	can (540 mL) mixed beans, drained and rinsed
1/2 cup	dried cranberries
3 tbsp	orange juice
2 tbsp	apple cider vinegar
1 tbsp	canola oil
1	small clove garlic, minced
2 tsp	Dijon mustard
1/4 tsp	each salt and pepper
1/4 cup	chopped fresh mint or flat-leaf parsley

1. In large pot of boiling water, cook wheat berries, covered, for about 1 hour or until tender but still slightly chewy. Drain and rinse under cold water until cool. Drain well and place in large bowl. Add apples, spinach, beans and cranberries.

2. In small bowl, whisk together orange juice, vinegar, oil, garlic, mustard, salt and pepper. Pour over wheat berry mixture and toss to coat. Add mint and stir to combine well.

Makes 6 to 8 servings.

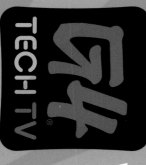

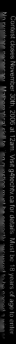

TUNA SALAD BOATS   GREEN-LIGHT

Canned tuna is a good source of protein and easy to prepare. It is also a popular request for lunch, so my advice
is to make it interesting and make it often.

1 cup	cooked chickpeas
2	cans (120 g each) chunk tuna packed in water, drained
½ cup	diced celery
½ cup	diced red bell pepper
1	dill pickle, finely diced
¼ cup	non-fat mayonnaise
2 tbsp	plain non-fat yogurt
1 tbsp	lemon juice
¼ tsp	each salt and pepper
4	small leaves Boston or radicchio lettuce
Quarter	cucumber, thinly sliced
1	tomato, cut in wedges

1. In bowl, using potato masher, mash chickpeas
   coarsely. Add tuna, celery, red pepper and pickle.
2. In small bowl, whisk together mayonnaise, yogurt,
   lemon juice, salt and pepper. Stir into tuna mixture.
   Divide mixture among lettuce leaves and garnish with
   cucumber slices and tomato wedges.

Makes 4 servings.

Meatless

VEGGIE BEAN BURGERS

Fibre-rich bean burgers are easy and inexpensive to make, highly nutritious and delicious.

1	can (540 mL) white kidney beans or lentils, drained and rinsed
1	egg
1/2 cup	wheat bran
1/4 cup	finely chopped almonds
2 tbsp	chopped fresh mint
1	small clove garlic, minced
1/4 tsp	each salt and pepper
2 tsp	canola oil

Coriander Yogurt Sauce:

1/4 cup	non-fat plain yogurt
1 tbsp	chopped fresh coriander
1/4 tsp	ground cumin
Pinch	salt

1. In large bowl, using potato masher, mash beans until smooth. Stir in egg, bran, almonds, mint, garlic, salt and pepper until well combined. Divide mixture into 4 equal portions and form into ½-inch-thick patties.

2. In large non-stick skillet, heat oil over medium heat. Cook patties for about 12 minutes, turning once, or until golden brown.

3. **Coriander Yogurt Sauce:** Meanwhile, in bowl, stir together yogurt, coriander, cumin and salt until combined. Dollop onto burgers before serving.

Makes 4 servings.

Helpful Hint: These burgers can be served on half a whole wheat bun with sliced tomatoes, cucumbers and lettuce.

BEAN TACOS

Serve these tacos with a variety of toppings, along with basmati rice and salad.

2 tsp	canola oil
1	onion, chopped
2	cloves garlic, minced
1	green bell pepper, diced
2 tsp	chili powder
1 tsp	paprika
1/2 tsp	ground cumin
2	cans (540 mL each) red kidney beans, drained and rinsed
1 cup	low-fat salsa
1	pkg (340 g) small whole wheat tortillas
1 1/2 cups	shredded romaine lettuce
2	tomatoes, diced
1/2 cup	non-fat sour cream

1. In large non-stick skillet, heat oil over medium heat. Cook onion, garlic, green pepper, chili powder, paprika and cumin for about 5 minutes or until softened.
2. Add beans and salsa and cook for about 5 minutes or until heated through. Using potato masher, mash about half of the bean mixture. Stir with remaining bean mixture to combine.
3. Divide bean mixture among tortillas and top with lettuce, tomatoes and sour cream. Roll up.

Makes 5 servings.

SOUTHWEST VEGGIE BAKE

There are many varieties of frozen mixed vegetables on the market, and using them makes this casserole easy to prepare. Look for colourful combinations of veggies.

2 cups	low-fat salsa
1/3 cup	liquid eggs
2 tbsp	chopped fresh coriander
2 tsp	dried oregano
1/2 tsp	ground cumin
Pinch	each salt and pepper
1	pkg (340 g) Veggie Ground Round
1	can (540 mL) black beans, drained and rinsed
2 1/2 cups	frozen mixed vegetables
1/2 cup	light-style Monterey Jack or colby cheese

1. In bowl, stir together salsa, liquid eggs, coriander, oregano, cumin, salt and pepper. Break up Veggie Ground Round and add to salsa mixture with black beans. Stir to combine; set aside.

2. Place vegetables in greased 8-inch casserole dish. Cover and microwave on High for 5 minutes. Drain any excess water and top with Veggie Ground Round mixture. Sprinkle with cheese. Cover with foil and bake in 400° F oven for about 30 minutes or until heated through.

Makes 4 to 6 servings.

ASIAN NOODLE STIR-FRY   GREEN-LIGHT

Mung bean noodles can be found in the international aisle of the supermarket. They come in little bundles or one large bundle. It is easiest to weigh the bundles for the correct amount, but each little bundle weighs approximately 1 ½ oz, which means you will need about 3 small bundles for this recipe.

4 oz	mung bean noodles
2 tsp	canola oil
1	onion, thinly sliced
1	carrot, thinly sliced
1	Asian eggplant, thinly sliced
1	red or green bell pepper, thinly sliced
2 cups	chopped broccoli
1 cup	chopped extra-firm tofu
½ cup	vegetable stock (low-fat, low-sodium)
¼ cup	orange juice
¼ cup	hoisin sauce
1 tbsp	chopped fresh ginger
½ tsp	Asian chili sauce or hot pepper flakes
⅓ cup	chopped roasted cashews

1. In large bowl, cover noodles with hot water and let stand for about 10 minutes or until softened. Drain and set aside.

2. In large non-stick skillet or wok, heat oil over medium-high heat. Stir-fry onion, carrot, eggplant, red pepper and broccoli for about 8 minutes or until softened

and beginning to turn golden. Add tofu and stir to combine.

3. Meanwhile, in bowl, whisk together stock, juice, hoisin sauce, ginger and chili sauce. Add noodles and stock mixture to skillet and toss to combine. Cook for about 3 minutes or until mixture has coated all the vegetables and noodles are hot. Sprinkle with cashews and serve.

Makes 4 servings.

Fish and Seafood

VEGETABLE-TOPPED FISH FILLETS

You can use salmon, tilapia, haddock or halibut fillets or steaks for this colourful dish.

2 tsp	extra-virgin olive oil
2 cups	quartered small mushrooms
1/2 cup	chopped red onion
2	cloves garlic, minced
2 cups	grape tomatoes, halved
1	zucchini, chopped
2 tbsp	each chopped fresh flat-leaf parsley and fresh basil
1/4 tsp	each salt and pepper
6	fish fillets, about 1 1/2 lb total
6	lemon wedges

1. In large non-stick skillet, heat oil over medium-high heat. Cook mushrooms, onion and garlic for about 5 minutes, or until beginning to turn golden. Add toma-

toes, zucchini, parsley, basil, salt and pepper. Cook for about 5 minutes, or until juices begin to form.

2. Place fillets on parchment paper–lined baking sheet. Top each fillet with vegetable mixture. Bake in 425° F oven for about 15 minutes or until fish flakes easily when tested with fork. Squeeze lemon wedge over each fillet before serving.

Makes 6 servings.

BROCCOLI-STUFFED SOLE   GREEN-LIGHT

These stuffed fish fillets are impressive enough to serve to company. For this recipe, thin fish fillets like tilapia or catfish work best.

1 tsp	canola oil
1	shallot, minced
2	cloves garlic, minced
1 cup	chopped broccoli
1 cup	cooked red kidney beans, chopped
1/4 cup	fish or vegetable stock, or water
1/4 cup	light garlic and herb cream cheese
2 tbsp	each chopped fresh flat-leaf parsley and fresh chives
6	sole fillets (about 1 1/2 lb total)
1/4 tsp	each salt and pepper

1. In non-stick skillet, heat oil over medium heat and cook shallot and garlic for 2 minutes. Add broccoli, kidney beans and stock. Cover and cook for about 3 minutes or until broccoli is tender-crisp. Stir in cream cheese, parsley and chives. Let cool slightly.

2. Spoon one-sixth of broccoli mixture in centre of each fillet. Roll up gently to cover filling and place in small baking pan. Sprinkle with salt and pepper. Bake in 425° F oven for about 15 minutes or until fish is cooked.

Makes 4 to 6 servings.

TERIYAKI FISH KEBABS   GREEN-LIGHT

These marinated fish kebabs are easy to make and festive. Serve them with basmati rice and baby bok choy.

¼ cup	soy sauce
1	green onion, minced
1 tsp	minced fresh ginger
1 tsp	Dijon mustard
1	small clove garlic, minced
1 ½ lb	halibut fillets, skinned
1	small zucchini, halved lengthwise
1 cup	small button mushrooms
2 tsp	toasted sesame oil
Pinch	pepper

1. In medium bowl, whisk together soy sauce, green onion, ginger, mustard and garlic; set aside. Cut fillets into 1 ½-inch pieces and add to soy mixture. Toss to coat and let marinate for 10 minutes.

2. Meanwhile, cut zucchini into ½-inch pieces and place in another bowl. Add mushrooms; drizzle with sesame oil and sprinkle with pepper. Toss to coat.

3. Skewer fish, zucchini and mushrooms alternately onto 6 metal or bamboo skewers. Place on greased grill over medium-high heat and grill for about 10 minutes, turning once, or until fish flakes easily when tested with fork, and vegetables are tender-crisp.

Makes 6 servings.

SALMON CAKES WITH TARRAGON TARTAR SAUCE

GREEN-LIGHT

These fish cakes are quick and easy, and a favourite of kids. Serve them alongside asparagus and carrots, or pack them into pitas with lettuce and tomato. Make mini salmon cakes for a great party appetizer.

2	cans (213 g) sockeye salmon, drained
1 cup	cooked white kidney beans
1	egg
¼ cup	finely diced red bell pepper
2	green onions, finely chopped
1	small clove garlic, minced
2 tbsp	chopped fresh flat-leaf parsley
Pinch	each salt and pepper
2 tsp	canola oil
2	whole wheat pita breads
2	tomatoes, sliced
1 ½ cups	shredded romaine lettuce

Tarragon Tartar Sauce:

¼ cup	non-fat mayonnaise
1 tbsp	lemon juice
1 tbsp	minced dill pickle
2 tsp	chopped fresh tarragon
Pinch	each salt and pepper

1. In large bowl, using potato masher, mash salmon and beans until well combined. Stir in egg, red pepper, green onions, garlic, parsley, salt and pepper until well combined. Divide mixture into 8 equal portions and form into ½-inch-thick patties.

2. In large non-stick skillet, heat oil over medium heat. Cook salmon cakes for about 10 minutes or until golden brown and crisp.

3. **Tarragon Tartar Sauce:** Meanwhile, in bowl, whisk together mayonnaise, lemon juice, pickle, tarragon, salt and pepper; set aside.

4. Cut pita breads in half and open pocket. Divide tomato and lettuce among pitas. Fill with salmon cakes and dollop with tartar sauce.

Makes 4 servings.

TUNA CASSEROLE   GREEN-LIGHT

This G.I.-friendly version of a traditional family favourite
uses whole wheat noodles and less cheese.

2 cups	whole wheat rotini pasta
2 cups	frozen California-style mixed vegetables
2 tbsp	canola oil
½ cup	finely chopped onion
1 tsp	dried thyme
½ tsp	dry mustard
¼ cup	whole wheat flour
2 cups	skim milk
¼ tsp	salt
Pinch	pepper
2	cans (120 g each) chunk tuna packed in water, drained
2 tbsp	grated Parmesan cheese

1. In large pot of boiling salted water, cook pasta for 7
   minutes. Add vegetables and cook for about 2 minutes
   or until pasta is al dente and vegetables are tender-
   crisp. Drain well and set aside.
2. Meanwhile, in saucepan, heat oil over medium heat.
   Cook onion, thyme and mustard for about 2 minutes
   or until softened. Add flour and cook, stirring, for 1
   minute. Slowly whisk in milk and continue cooking,
   whisking gently, for about 5 minutes or until mixture
   coats back of spoon. Remove from heat and stir in salt
   and pepper.

3. Add cooked pasta and vegetables and tuna. Stir to combine well. Scrape into 6-cup casserole dish and sprinkle with cheese. Bake in 375° F oven for about 15 minutes or until bubbly and heated through.

Makes 4 servings.

Salmon Option: Use 2 cans (213 g each) canned salmon instead of tuna.

Crab Option: Use 1 pkg (7 oz) frozen crab, thawed and drained, instead of tuna.

SALMON PASTA

For days when you can't get to the market for fresh salmon, use 2 cans of salmon or tuna instead.

2 tsp	canola oil
1	small onion, finely chopped
2	cloves garlic, minced
2 cups	chicken or fish stock
1 cup	whole wheat macaroni pasta
1 ½ cups	chopped broccoli
⅓ cup	light herb and garlic cream cheese
1	salmon fillet, skinned (about 6 oz)
2 tbsp	chopped fresh flat-leaf parsley
Pinch	each salt and pepper

1. In saucepan, heat 1 tsp of the oil over medium heat. Cook onion and garlic for about 3 minutes or until softened. Add chicken stock and bring to boil. Add pasta and cover; reduce heat to simmer and cook for 10 minutes. Stir in broccoli and cream cheese. Remove from heat. Let stand, covered, for 10 minutes.

2. Rub remaining oil over fillet and sprinkle with parsley, salt and pepper. Roast in small baking pan in 425° F oven for about 10 minutes. Break up salmon into chunks and add to pasta mixture. Stir gently to combine.

Makes 2 servings.

LINGUINE WITH CLAMS

GREEN-LIGHT

A staple at most Italian restaurants, this rich-tasting pasta dish is easy to make for family dinners.

2 tsp	extra-virgin olive oil
1	onion, chopped
4	cloves garlic, minced
2 tsp	dried oregano
1 tsp	dried basil
1/4 tsp	hot pepper flakes
1	can (796 mL) diced tomatoes
1	zucchini, chopped
2	cans (142 g each) baby clams, drained and rinsed
1/4 cup	chopped fresh flat-leaf parsley
1/4 tsp	pepper
Pinch	salt
6 oz	whole wheat spaghetti or linguine

1. In saucepan, heat oil over medium heat. Cook onion, garlic, oregano, basil and hot pepper flakes for about 5 minutes or until softened. Add tomatoes and zucchini and bring to boil. Reduce heat and simmer for 10 minutes. Add clams, parsley, pepper and salt and cook, stirring, for about 10 minutes or until thickened.
2. Meanwhile, in large pot of boiling salted water, cook pasta for about 8 minutes or until al dente. Drain and divide among 4 plates. Top pasta with clam sauce.

Makes 4 servings.

Poultry

OPEN-FACED LUNCH SANDWICH

This delicious sandwich is chock full of protein and vegetables. For a change, substitute the bread with pita halves.

4	slices 100% stone-ground whole wheat bread
Half	ripe avocado
1/2 cup	cooked chickpeas, chopped
1/4 cup	Light Boursin or La Vache Qui Rit (The Laughing Cow) Light cheese
2 tbsp	chopped fresh basil or flat-leaf parsley
1/4 tsp	each salt and pepper
4	slices lean turkey (optional)
1 cup	chopped cucumber
1	plum tomato, chopped
1/4 cup	grated carrot
1 tbsp	red wine vinegar
1/4 tsp	dried oregano

1. Place the bread slices in the toaster or under broiler to toast bread.
2. In bowl, using fork, mash avocado until almost smooth. Add chickpeas, cheese, parsley and half each of the salt and pepper. Divide and spread over bread. Top with turkey, if using.
3. In bowl, combine cucumber, tomato, carrot, vinegar, oregano and remaining salt and pepper. Divide evenly over toast.

Makes 2 servings.

Tuna Option: Omit turkey and add 1 can (120 g) water-packed tuna to cucumber mixture to serve on bread or in pita.

STUFFED PORTOBELLO MUSHROOMS GREEN-LIGHT

These meaty mushrooms are a novel and tasty alternative to stuffed peppers.

1 tsp	canola oil
12 oz	lean ground turkey or chicken
1	onion, finely chopped
2	cloves garlic, minced
1 tsp	dried oregano
1/2 tsp	dried basil
Pinch	hot pepper flakes (optional)
2 cups	lightly packed baby spinach
1/2 cup	chopped roasted red pepper
1/2 tsp	salt
1/4 tsp	pepper
1/2 cup	wheat bran
1/4 cup	liquid egg whites
4	portobello mushrooms
2 tbsp	grated Parmesan cheese

1. In non-stick skillet, heat oil over medium-high heat. Cook turkey, breaking up with back of spoon, for about 8 minutes or until no longer pink inside. Drain fat, if necessary. Add onion, garlic, oregano, basil, and hot pepper flakes, if using, and cook for about 5 minutes or until onion is softened. Transfer to bowl and add spinach, roasted red pepper, salt and pepper. Let cool slightly. Add bran and egg whites and stir to combine.

2. Remove stems of mushrooms and scrape out dark gills from underside using small spoon. Place on parchment paper–lined baking sheet. Divide turkey mixture evenly over scraped side of mushrooms. Sprinkle with cheese and bake in 400° F oven for about 15 minutes or until mushrooms are tender.

Makes 4 servings.

Sun-Dried Tomato Option: Omit roasted red pepper and use ¼ cup sun-dried tomatoes, soaked in boiling water and drained. Chop and add to filling.

Vegetarian Option: Substitute Veggie Ground Round for the ground turkey. You can substitute 2 egg whites for the ¼ cup liquid egg whites.

Helpful Hint: To clean mushrooms, use a damp paper towel. Do not rinse or soak as they will absorb the water.

CHICKEN FRIED RICE

GREEN-LIGHT

Chinese fried rice is generally high in fat and low in protein and fibre. This low-G.I. version is loaded with chicken and colourful vegetables, and won't leave you feeling hungry again soon after eating it.

1 1/2 cups	chicken stock (low-fat, low-sodium)
3/4 cup	brown rice
Pinch	salt
1 tsp	sesame oil
2	boneless skinless chicken breasts, chopped
1 cup	sliced mushrooms
1	green onion, chopped
2	carrots, diced
1/2 cup	sliced celery
1 cup	cooked chickpeas
1/4 cup	light soy sauce
2 cups	bean sprouts

1. In saucepan, bring 1 1/4 cups of the chicken stock, rice and salt to boil. Reduce heat to low, cover and cook for about 25 minutes or until liquid is absorbed. Fluff with fork and set aside.

2. In large non-stick skillet, heat oil over medium-high heat. Cook chicken and mushrooms for about 8 minutes or until chicken is no longer pink inside. Add green onions, carrot, celery, chickpeas and cooked rice. Cook, stirring, for 2 minutes to combine.

3. Add remaining chicken stock and soy sauce and cook for 5 minutes. Add bean sprouts and toss to combine.

Makes 4 servings.

Vegetarian Fried Rice Option: Substitute vegetable stock for the chicken stock. Substitute 1 ½ cups chopped extra-firm tofu for the chicken.

Egg Option: Omit chicken and use ¾ cup liquid eggs. In non-stick skillet, heat 1 tsp canola oil over medium heat and scramble egg for about 2 minutes or until no longer runny. Add to rice mixture with bean sprouts.

Helpful Hint: You can use 1 ½ cups of leftover cooked rice and 2 cups of leftover cooked chicken.

CHICKEN CHOP SUEY   GREEN-LIGHT

It's easy to make this perennial Chinese takeout favourite low-G.I. If you prefer, use a can of sliced water chestnuts instead of the bamboo shoots.

1 lb	boneless skinless chicken breasts
2 tsp	canola oil
4	green onions, sliced
1	stalk celery, thinly sliced
1	carrot, thinly sliced
2 cups	sliced mushrooms
3/4 cup	chicken stock (low-fat, low-sodium)
2 tbsp	light soy sauce
1 tbsp	cornstarch
2 cups	bean sprouts
1	can (227 mL) sliced bamboo shoots, drained and rinsed
1 tbsp	chopped fresh ginger

1. Thinly slice chicken crosswise into bite-sized pieces; set aside.

2. In large non-stick skillet or wok, heat half of the oil over medium-high heat. Cook chicken, stirring constantly, for about 8 minutes or until no longer pink inside. Transfer to plate. Add remaining oil to skillet and cook green onions, celery, carrot and mushrooms, stirring occasionally, for about 5 minutes or until vegetables are tender-crisp. Return chicken to skillet.

3. Meanwhile, in small bowl, whisk together chicken stock, soy sauce and cornstarch. Pour into skillet along with bean sprouts, bamboo shoots and ginger. Cook, stirring, for about 2 minutes or until sauce is thickened and bubbly.

Makes 4 servings.

Tofu Option: Omit chicken. Use 1 lb extra-firm tofu, thinly sliced, and toss with 1 tsp toasted sesame oil; sauté quickly. Continue with recipe.

GARLIC LIME CHICKEN

GREEN-LIGHT

The addition of lime gives this chicken a tropical flavour.
Serve it with roasted vegetables and rice to complete the
meal.

6	cloves garlic, minced
1 tbsp	grated lime rind
3 tbsp	lime juice
1 tbsp	canola oil
2 tsp	chili powder
1/2 tsp	each salt and pepper
1 1/2 lb	boneless skinless chicken thighs
12	mini new red potatoes
3	green or orange bell peppers
2 tbsp	chopped fresh coriander or flat-leaf parsley

1. In large shallow dish, whisk together garlic, lime rind
   and juice, half of the oil, chili powder and half each of
   the salt and pepper. Add chicken and turn to coat.
   Cover and refrigerate for 30 minutes.

2. Meanwhile, cut potatoes in half and place in large
   bowl. Cut green peppers in half and remove ribs and
   seeds. Cut into thick slices and add to bowl. Toss with
   remaining oil, salt and pepper.

3. Remove chicken from marinade and place in centre of
   large parchment paper–lined baking sheet. Place potatoes and peppers around edge of chicken and roast in
   425° F oven for about 35 minutes or until chicken is no

longer pink inside and potatoes are tender. Sprinkle with coriander.

Makes 4 servings.

OVEN-FRIED CHICKEN LEGS YELLOW-LIGHT

Everyone loves fried chicken, but surprise, surprise: it's loaded with fat. The good news is that by using crunchy high-fibre cereal and roasting the chicken in the oven, you can have G.I.-friendly fried chicken. Enjoy!

2 cups	bran flakes
1 tbsp	grated Parmesan cheese
1/2 tsp	Italian herb seasoning
Pinch	each salt and pepper
3 tbsp	Dijon mustard
10	skinless chicken drumsticks (about 1 1/2 lb)

1. Place bran flakes in resealable plastic bag and finely crush to make 1 ¼ cups. Add cheese, Italian herb seasoning, salt and pepper and shake to combine. Pour bran mixture onto waxed paper or shallow dish.

2. Spread mustard evenly over drumsticks and roll in bran flake mixture. Place on parchment paper–lined baking sheet and bake in 400° F oven for about 40 minutes or until chicken is no longer pink inside.

Makes 4 to 5 servings.

Chicken Strip Option: Omit chicken drumsticks and use 4 boneless skinless chicken breasts. For strips, cut each breast into ½-inch-thick strips lengthwise; toss with mustard and coat with bran mixture. Bake in 400° F oven for about 15 minutes.

Chicken Nugget Option: Omit chicken drumsticks and use 4 boneless skinless chicken breasts. For nuggets, cut each breast into ¾-inch-cubes; toss with mustard and coat with bran mixture. Bake in 400° F oven for about 12 minutes.

Buttermilk Mustard Dipping Sauce: In bowl, whisk together ¼ cup buttermilk, 2 tbsp Dijon mustard, 1 tsp sugar substitute and 1 tsp minced chives. Serve with strips or nuggets.

Pork Option: You can substitute pork loin for the chicken breasts.

Herb Option: Omit Italian herb seasoning and substitute either dried oregano, thyme or basil.

ORANGE CHICKEN WITH NUTS

Fans of sweet-and-sour dishes will enjoy this orange-flavoured chicken. The almonds add calcium to this Asian-influenced meal.

2	oranges
1 tbsp	canola oil
2	boneless skinless chicken breasts, chopped
2 tsp	minced fresh ginger
1/4 tsp	each salt and pepper
2	green onions, chopped
1	each red and green bell peppers, chopped
Pinch	hot pepper flakes
1/4 cup	chicken stock (low-fat, low-sodium)
3 tbsp	soy sauce
2 tsp	cornstarch
1/2 cup	sliced almonds, toasted
	Basmati rice (see recipe on next page)

1. Using rasp or grater, remove 1 tsp of the orange rind and set aside. Cut away orange rind and pith from 1 of the oranges and discard. Chop orange flesh coarsely. Cut other orange in half and squeeze out juice; set aside.

2. In large non-stick skillet or wok, heat half of the oil over medium-high heat. Cook chicken, ginger and a pinch each of the salt and pepper for about 6 minutes or until chicken is no longer pink inside. Transfer to plate. Add remaining oil to skillet and cook green

onions, red and green peppers and hot pepper flakes, stirring constantly, for about 6 minutes or until tender-crisp.

3. In small bowl, whisk together chicken stock, soy sauce, reserved orange rind and juice, cornstarch and remaining salt and pepper. Add chicken, chopped orange and sauce to skillet and cook, stirring, for about 5 minutes or until sauce is thickened and chicken and vegetables are coated. Sprinkle with almonds and serve with rice.

Makes 2 servings.

Cooked Basmati Rice: In small saucepan, combine 1 ½ cups water, ¾ cup basmati rice and pinch each salt and pepper and bring to boil. Reduce heat to low, cover and cook for about 10 minutes or until rice is tender and water is absorbed. Stir in 2 tbsp chopped fresh flat-leaf parsley.

Pork Option: Substitute 1 small pork tenderloin, chopped, for the chicken.

Tofu Option: Substitute 1 pkg (350 g) extra-firm tofu, chopped, for the chicken.

TURKEY MEAT LOAF

GREEN-LIGHT

Meat loaf is a lifesaver for most families since it suits almost everyone's tastes. To please the kids and speed up the cooking time, try the mini-muffin variation.

1 tsp	canola oil
2 cups	chopped mushrooms
1	onion, finely chopped
4	cloves garlic, minced
1 tsp	dried thyme
¼ tsp	each salt and pepper
¾ cup	low-fat pasta sauce
½ cup	wheat bran
1	egg
¼ cup	chopped fresh flat-leaf parsley
1 tbsp	Worcestershire sauce
1 ½ lb	lean ground turkey or chicken

1. In non-stick skillet, heat oil over medium heat and cook mushrooms, onion, garlic, thyme, salt and pepper for about 8 minutes or until softened and liquid evaporates from mushrooms. Transfer to bowl; let cool slightly.

2. Stir ¼ cup of the pasta sauce into mushroom mixture. Add bran, egg, parsley and Worcestershire sauce and combine well. Using hands, mix in turkey to combine evenly. Pack mixture into 8- x 4-inch loaf pan and spread remaining pasta sauce evenly on top. Bake in 350° F oven for about 1 hour or until meat thermometer

registers 160° F when inserted in centre of meat loaf. Let cool slightly before serving.

Makes 6 servings.

Mini-Muffin Option: Pack turkey mixture into 12 muffin cups and spread with remaining pasta sauce. Bake for about 35 minutes or until meat thermometer registers 160° F when inserted in centre.

Ground Beef Option: Substitute extra-lean ground beef for the turkey.

Bell Pepper Option: Substitute 1 large red or green bell pepper, diced, for the chopped mushrooms.

Meat

RIGATONI WITH MINI-MEATBALLS GREEN-LIGHT

For busy families, a little meal preplanning always helps during the week. This hearty casserole can be made ahead of time and frozen for another day.

8 oz	lean ground chicken or turkey
2 tbsp	chopped fresh Italian parsley
1	large clove garlic, minced
1 tsp	salt
Pinch	pepper
1 tbsp	extra-virgin olive oil
1	onion, chopped
2 cups	chopped eggplant
1	zucchini, chopped
1	small carrot, finely chopped
1 tbsp	dried oregano
2	cans plum tomatoes (796 mL each), puréed
½ cup	cooked red kidney beans
3 cups	rigatoni pasta
2 tbsp	grated Parmesan cheese

1. In bowl, mix together chicken, parsley, garlic, pinch of the salt and pepper until well combined. Using wet hands, roll 1 heaping tsp of the mixture into a small meatball and place on parchment paper–lined baking sheet. Repeat with remaining mixture. Bake in 350° F oven for about 8 minutes or until no longer pink inside.

2. Meanwhile, in large saucepan, heat oil over medium-high heat. Cook onion and eggplant for about 8 minutes or until golden and softened. Reduce heat to medium and add zucchini, carrot and oregano. Cook, stirring, for about 5 minutes or until softened. Add puréed tomatoes and remaining salt; bring to boil. Add cooked meatballs and beans; reduce heat and simmer for about 30 minutes or until slightly thickened.

3. Meanwhile, in large pot of boiling salted water, cook rigatoni for about 10 minutes or until al dente. Drain and add to meatballs and sauce; stir to combine. Pour into shallow casserole dish and sprinkle with cheese.

Makes 4 to 6 servings.

Helpful Hint: To make this dish ahead, pour the mixture into a casserole dish and let cool for about 30 minutes before covering and refrigerating for up to 1 day. Or freeze for up to 2 weeks. Let thaw in refrigerator before reheating in 325° F oven for about 45 minutes or until bubbly and knife inserted in centre comes out hot. Sprinkle with cheese before reheating.

Tip: Purée plum tomatoes in blender or food processor.

LEAN CHUNKY BEEF CHILI   GREEN-LIGHT

Using chopped beef instead of ground beef gives chili a chunkier texture. Raid your pantry for whatever beans you have on hand, and be sure to add lots of veggies for more taste and nutrition.

2 lb	eye of round roast
2 tsp	canola oil
1	large onion, chopped
3	cloves garlic, minced
1	stalk celery, chopped
1	carrot, chopped
2 cups	sliced mushrooms
1 tbsp	chili powder
1 tbsp	dried oregano
2 tsp	ground cumin
1	can (796 mL) diced tomatoes
1 ½ cups	beef stock
¼ cup	tomato paste
1	can (540 mL) chickpeas, drained and rinsed
1	can (540 mL) red kidney beans, drained and rinsed

1. Cut roast into ½-inch-thick slices. Cut each slice into ½-inch strips and then into ½-inch cubes.
2. In large shallow saucepan, heat half of the oil over medium-high heat. Brown meat in batches, adding more oil as necessary. Transfer to plate. Add onion, garlic, celery, carrot, mushrooms, chili powder, oregano

and cumin. Cook, stirring, for about 10 minutes or until vegetables are softened.

3. Add tomatoes, stock and tomato paste and bring to boil. Add beef and simmer for about 45 minutes or until beef is tender. Add chickpeas and kidney beans; cover and cook for about 15 minutes or until thickened.

Makes 6 to 8 servings.

Ground Meat Option: You can substitute extra-lean ground beef, veal, turkey or chicken for the beef cubes.

OPEN-FACED MEATBALL SUBS   GREEN-LIGHT

Here's a sandwich hearty enough for dinner. The meatballs can be made with turkey, beef or chicken.

12 oz	ground turkey or extra-lean ground beef
⅓ cup	wheat bran
¼ cup	chopped fresh flat-leaf parsley
1	egg
1	clove garlic, minced
¼ tsp	each salt and pepper
1 tsp	canola oil
8 oz	mushrooms, thinly sliced
1	green bell pepper, chopped (optional)
½ tsp	dried oregano
1	jar (700 mL) low-fat chunky vegetable pasta sauce
2	whole wheat sub buns, halved lengthwise
1 cup	shredded romaine lettuce
½ cup	shredded light-style mozzarella cheese

1. In large bowl, mix together turkey, bran, parsley, egg,
    garlic, salt and pepper. Using hands, form mixture into
    1-inch meatballs and place on parchment paper– or
    foil-lined baking sheet. Bake in 350° F oven for about 15
    minutes or until no longer pink inside.

2. Meanwhile, in non-stick skillet, heat oil over medium-
    high heat. Cook mushrooms, green pepper and
    oregano for about 8 minutes or until golden and liquid
    evaporates from mushrooms. Transfer to plate.

3. Add pasta sauce to same skillet and heat over medium heat. Add cooked meatballs and bring to simmer. Cook, stirring occasionally, for about 5 minutes or until meatballs are well coated.
4. Hollow out inside of buns, leaving ¼ inch around edge. Divide lettuce, cheese and mushrooms and pepper mixture among sub buns. Top with meatballs and sauce.

Makes 4 servings.

Storage Option: You can freeze the meatballs after cooking and cooling; after thawing, reheat them in the sauce for a quick evening meal.

Helpful Hint: These meatballs can also be eaten without the bun, with the peppers and mushrooms and pasta sauce.

HAMBURGERS FOR EVERYONE

Make these burgers year-round either on your grill or in a skillet. Remember to use only half a bun per serving. To make your burgers even more green-light, forget the bun and serve the patties with vegetables.

1	small onion, grated
2	cloves garlic, minced
1/4 cup	minced celery
1/4 cup	fresh whole wheat bread crumbs
1	egg
1 tbsp	Dijon mustard
2 tsp	Worcestershire sauce
Pinch	each salt and pepper
1 lb	extra-lean ground beef, turkey or chicken

Quick Coleslaw:

2 cups	shredded coleslaw mix
2 tbsp	white wine vinegar
2 tsp	canola oil
1/2 tsp	celery seed
1/4 tsp	salt

2	whole wheat hamburger buns
1	tomato, sliced

1. In large bowl, combine onion, garlic, celery, bread crumbs, egg, mustard, Worcestershire sauce, salt and pepper. Add beef and, using hands, combine well. Divide mixture into 4 equal mounds.

2. Shape each mound into ½-inch-thick hamburger patties and place on greased grill over medium-high heat. Cook, turning once, for about 12 minutes or until no longer pink inside.

3. **Quick Coleslaw:** In bowl, combine coleslaw mix, vinegar, oil, celery seed and salt; set aside.

4. Divide hamburger buns among 4 plates and top with hamburgers. Divide tomato slices among hamburgers and top with coleslaw mixture.

Makes 4 servings.

Helpful Hint: Coleslaw mix is available in the produce aisle, where you find other types of salad in bags. It does not contain any dressing. It is usually a mixture of green and red cabbage with some shredded carrot. If this is unavailable, finely shred about ¼ of a small green cabbage.

Skillet Option: To cook hamburgers in a skillet or grill pan, cook over medium-high heat for about 15 minutes, turning once.

FRENCH ONION PORK MEDALLIONS   GREEN-LIGHT

In this dish, French onion soup is transformed into a
rich, flavourful sauce for pork.

1	pork tenderloin (about 1 lb)
2 tsp	chopped fresh rosemary (or ½ tsp dried)
¼ tsp	each salt and pepper
2 tsp	canola oil
2	large onions, thinly sliced
1	red bell pepper, thinly sliced
2	cloves garlic, minced
1 ½ cups	beef stock
1 tbsp	Worcestershire sauce

1. Trim all fat from the tenderloin, and cut into 1-inch
   medallions. Sprinkle with rosemary and half each of
   the salt and pepper.
2. In large non-stick skillet, heat half of the oil over
   medium-high heat. Brown pork and transfer to plate.
   Return skillet to heat and add remaining oil. Cook
   onions, stirring, for about 18 minutes or until very soft
   and golden. Add red pepper and garlic and cook for 2
   minutes.
3. Add stock, Worcestershire sauce and remaining salt
   and pepper and bring to boil. Boil for 5 minutes.
   Return pork to skillet and cook for about 2 minutes.

Makes 4 servings.

MUSHROOM AND GRAVY PORK CHOPS

Nothing turns food into comfort food better than gravy. For a change, substitute chicken for pork chops.

1 tsp	Italian herb seasoning
½ tsp	each dried basil, salt and pepper
4	boneless pork loin chops
2 tsp	extra-virgin olive oil
1	large onion, thinly sliced
1 lb	mushrooms, sliced
1 tbsp	chopped fresh thyme (or 1 tsp dried)
2 tbsp	whole wheat flour
1 cup	chicken stock (low-fat, low-sodium)

1. In small bowl, combine Italian herb seasoning, dried basil and half each of the salt and pepper. Sprinkle evenly on both sides of pork chops.

2. In large non-stick skillet, heat oil over medium-high heat. Brown chops on both sides; transfer to plate. Add onion, mushrooms, thyme and remaining salt and pepper. Cook, stirring, for 10 minutes. Sprinkle with flour and cook, stirring, for 1 minute. Pour in stock and bring to boil. Boil gently for about 3 minutes or until slightly thickened. Return pork chops to skillet and cook, turning occasionally, for about 5 minutes or until just a hint of pink remains inside pork.

Makes 4 servings.

ROASTED GARLIC PORK TENDERLOIN GREEN-LIGHT WITH MIXED BEAN TOSS

Roasting pungent garlic magically transforms it into a sweet, rich treat. This recipe can easily be doubled for entertaining.

1	head garlic
1 tbsp	Dijon mustard
2 tsp	chopped fresh thyme (or ½ tsp dried)
½ tsp	black pepper
2 tsp	canola oil
1	pork tenderloin (about 1 lb)

Mixed Bean Toss:

1	can (540 mL) mixed beans, drained and rinsed
3 tbsp	chopped fresh basil or flat-leaf parsley
4 tsp	apple cider vinegar
2 tsp	canola oil
Pinch	each salt and pepper

1. Wrap garlic in small piece of foil and roast in 400° F oven for about 35 minutes or until soft when squeezed. Let cool slightly. Squeeze garlic into bowl and mash with fork to form paste. Stir in mustard, thyme and pepper; set aside.

2. In non-stick skillet, heat oil over medium-high heat. Brown tenderloin on all sides. Transfer to small parchment paper–lined baking sheet and spread with

roasted garlic mixture. Roast in 425° F oven for about 20 minutes or until just a hint of pink remains inside pork. Let stand for 5 minutes before slicing thinly.

3. **Mixed Bean Toss:** Meanwhile, in bowl, stir together beans, basil, vinegar, oil, salt and pepper until combined. Serve with pork.

Makes 4 servings.

Helpful Hint: You can roast a few heads of garlic at a time and refrigerate or freeze them. Warm them in the microwave before squeezing.

Snacks

CHEESE AND NUT SPREAD

GREEN-LIGHT

This spread makes a delicious snack, or appetizer for dinner parties. The nuts give it a delightfully crunchy texture. Serve it with carrots, celery sticks, cucumber slices or whole wheat pita triangles.

1 cup	non-fat cottage cheese
1/2 cup	shredded light-style Cheddar cheese
1 cup	finely shredded baby spinach leaves
2 tbsp	finely chopped carrots
2 tbsp	finely chopped green onion
1	small clove garlic, minced
2 tsp	Dijon mustard
1/2 tsp	dried basil
1/4 tsp	each salt and pepper
3 tbsp	chopped toasted almonds*

1. In bowl, stir together cottage and Cheddar cheeses, spinach, carrots, green onion, garlic, mustard, basil, salt and pepper until well combined. Scrape into serving bowl and sprinkle with almonds. Cover and refrigerate for at least 15 minutes before serving. Spread may be refrigerated for up to 2 days. Be sure to stir up the mixture before serving.

Makes about 1 ²/₃ cups.

* **Toasting Almonds:** Place almonds on baking sheet and bake in 350° F oven for about 8 minutes or until fragrant. Remove from baking sheet and let cool. Chop if necessary.

SOYBEAN HUMMUS

GREEN-LIGHT

There are many variations of hummus, a popular Middle Eastern dip. This one uses green soybeans, also known as *edamame*. You can find them fresh in the produce department of your supermarket, or frozen.

2 cups	shelled soybeans
2 tbsp	extra-virgin olive oil
2 tbsp	lemon juice
2 tbsp	water
1	small clove garlic, minced
1/2 tsp	ground cumin
1/4 tsp	salt
Pinch	pepper

1. In food processor, purée soybeans, olive oil, lemon juice and water until smooth. Pulse in garlic, cumin, salt and pepper until combined.

Makes about 2 cups.

Spicy Option: For a spicier version of hummus, add ½ tsp Asian chili paste along with garlic.

HOMEMADE APPLE AND PEAR SAUCE   GREEN-LIGHT

Served warm or cold, this variation on applesauce makes a nutritious snack. It also makes a wonderful addition to your kids' lunch boxes.

1 lb	cooking apples, cored and quartered
1 lb	Bartlett pears, cored and quartered
1/2 cup	pear nectar
1/3 cup	sugar substitute
1/2 tsp	ground cinnamon

1. In large saucepan, combine apples, pears, pear nectar, sugar substitute and cinnamon; bring to boil. Cover, reduce heat and simmer for about 10 minutes or until tender. Let cool slightly.
2. Scrape into blender or food processor and purée until smooth. Once it has cooled, it can be refrigerated for up to one week.

Makes about 2 ½ cups.

Helpful Hint: If you like a chunkier texture, simply pulse the mixture until desired texture is reached.

APPLESAUCE BARS

Perfect for picnics and lunch boxes, applesauce bars can be made ahead of time and frozen.

1 1/4 cups	whole wheat flour
1/2 cup	wheat bran
1/4 cup	ground flax
3/4 cup	brown sugar substitute
1 tbsp	baking powder
2 tsp	cinnamon
1/2 tsp	baking soda
1/2 tsp	ground nutmeg
Pinch	ground cloves
Pinch	salt
2 cups	Homemade Apple and Pear Sauce (see recipe, page 271)
2/3 cup	liquid eggs
1/3 cup	canola oil

1. In large bowl, whisk together flour, bran, flax, sugar substitute, baking powder, cinnamon, baking soda, nutmeg, cloves and salt. In another bowl, whisk together Apple and Pear Sauce, liquid eggs and oil; pour over flour mixture and stir until moistened.

2. Scrape batter into greased and parchment paper–lined 13- x 9-inch baking pan and bake in 350° F oven for about 30 minutes or until cake tester inserted in centre comes out clean. Let cool completely. These can be

covered and refrigerated for up to 3 days, or frozen for up to 2 weeks.

Makes 24 bars.

Nut Option: You can add ¾ cup chopped almonds or pecans to the batter before baking.

REFRIGERATOR RAISIN BRAN MUFFINS

Not many people have time to make muffins on a week-day morning, but if you already have the batter in the fridge, all you have do is scoop and bake. In just twenty minutes, you can have instant fresh muffins for your morning snack.

2 cups	All-Bran cereal
1 1/2 cups	boiling water
1 1/2 cups	whole wheat flour
1 cup	wheat bran
3/4 cup	sugar substitute
2 tbsp	baking powder
2 tsp	cinnamon
1/2 tsp	salt
2 cups	skim milk
2	eggs
1/4 cup	canola oil
1/4 cup	unsweetened applesauce or Homemade Apple and Pear Sauce (see recipe, page 271)
2 tsp	grated orange rind
1/2 cup	raisins

1. In bowl, combine cereal and boiling water. Let stand for 2 minutes and stir to soften.
2. In large bowl, whisk together flour, bran, sugar substitute, baking powder, cinnamon and salt.

3. In another bowl, whisk together milk, eggs, oil, apple-sauce and orange rind. Stir into bran mixture. Pour over flour mixture and stir until moistened. Add raisins and stir to combine. Cover and refrigerate for up to 2 days.

4. Gently stir batter before scooping into desired number of greased or paper-lined muffin tins. Bake in 400° F oven for about 20 minutes or until golden and firm to the touch.

Makes 24 small or 16 large muffins.

Dried Fruit Option: You can substitute dried chopped apples, dried cranberries or currants for the raisins.

Helpful Hint: Bake only as many muffins as you will need over the course of two days so you always have a fresh batch.

RHUBARB PEAR MUFFINS

Though rhubarb is best fresh in the summer, you can buy it frozen all year round and use it to make muffins, cakes and compotes. If you find the rhubarb too tart, simply sweeten it with a sugar substitute.

1 cup	All-Bran or 100% Bran cereal
3/4 cup	wheat bran
1 cup	buttermilk
1 cup	whole wheat flour
1/2 cup	brown sugar substitute
2 tsp	baking powder
1 tsp	grated lemon rind
1/4 tsp	baking soda
Pinch	salt
1/2 cup	liquid eggs
1/4 cup	canola oil
1 tsp	vanilla
1	ripe pear, cored and diced
1 1/2 cups	chopped fresh or frozen rhubarb

Streusel Topping:

1/4 cup	whole wheat flour
3 tbsp	brown sugar substitute
2 tbsp	soft non-hydrogenated margarine
1/2 tsp	cinnamon

1. In bowl, combine All-Bran and wheat bran. Pour over buttermilk and stir to combine; let stand for 10 minutes.

2. Meanwhile, whisk together flour, sugar substitute, baking powder, lemon rind, baking soda and salt. In another bowl, whisk together liquid eggs, oil and vanilla. Stir into bran mixture. Pour over flour mixture and stir to combine. Gently stir in pear and rhubarb until just combined.

3. Divide batter among 12 greased or paper-lined muffin tins.

4. **Streusel Topping:** In small bowl, combine whole wheat flour, sugar substitute, margarine and cinnamon until crumbly. Sprinkle over top of muffin batter and bake in 400° F oven for about 20 minutes or until golden and firm to the touch.

Makes 12 muffins.

Storage: Wrap each muffin individually in plastic wrap and freeze in airtight container for up to 2 weeks or refrigerate for up to 2 days.

OATMEAL CRANBERRY SCONES   GREEN-LIGHT

Enjoy these scones with some cottage cheese and fresh fruit for a morning snack or late-afternoon pick-me-up.

1 ¼ cups	whole wheat flour
½ cup	wheat bran
2 tbsp	sugar substitute
2 tsp	baking powder
¼ tsp	ground nutmeg
Pinch	ground cloves
½ cup	soft non-hydrogenated margarine
1 cup	large-flake rolled oats
½ cup	chopped dried cranberries
⅓ cup	skim milk
¼ cup	liquid eggs

1. In bowl, combine flour, bran, sugar substitute, baking powder, nutmeg and cloves. Using fingers, rub margarine into flour mixture until mixture resembles coarse crumbs. Using fork, stir in oats and cranberries.

2. In small bowl, whisk together ¼ cup of the milk and liquid eggs. Pour over flour mixture and stir until just moistened. Turn out dough onto floured surface and pat into 8-inch round. Cut into 12 wedges. Place on parchment paper–lined baking sheet and brush tops with remaining milk. Bake in 425° F oven for about 12 minutes or until golden brown.

Makes 12 scones.

Desserts

FROZEN RICOTTA TREAT

GREEN-LIGHT

This is a delightful weekday dessert.

1	tub (500 g) light ricotta cheese
¼ cup	sugar substitute
1 tbsp	vanilla
1 ½ cups	frozen wild blueberries
1 cup	chopped fresh strawberries
1 cup	non-fat sugar-free strawberry yogurt
1 tbsp	chopped fresh mint

1. In food processor, purée ricotta cheese, sugar substitute and vanilla until smooth. Scrape into bowl and stir in blueberries and strawberries; set aside.
2. Line 8- x 4-inch loaf pan with plastic wrap and scrape ricotta mixture into pan, smoothing top. Cover top with plastic wrap and freeze for about 4 hours or until firm.
3. To serve, cut into 1-inch slices; dollop each with yogurt and sprinkle with mint.

Makes 8 servings.

GELATIN FRUIT DESSERT GREEN-LIGHT

Jiggly gelatin desserts are definitely kid-friendly. You can easily add variety by using different kinds of fruit.

½ cup	water
1	pkg (7 g) unflavoured gelatin
1 cup	unsweetened cranberry juice
⅓ cup	sugar substitute
1 cup	non-fat sugar-free plain yogurt
1	can (14 oz) sliced peaches, no sugar added, drained
1 cup	red seedless grapes

1. Pour water into small saucepan and sprinkle gelatin over top; let stand for 1 minute. Place over medium heat and stir until gelatin is melted. Add cranberry juice and sugar substitute and stir until combined. Refrigerate for about 1 hour, stirring occasionally, until thickened to consistency of egg whites. Stir in yogurt until combined.

2. Meanwhile, chop peaches coarsely and cut grapes in half lengthwise. Stir into gelatin mixture. Pour evenly into each of four 1-cup ramekins or shallow glass dishes and refrigerate for about 2 hours or until firm.

Makes 4 servings.

PEANUT BUTTER CRUNCH COOKIES   YELLOW-LIGHT

These crunchy and nutritious cookies are a great way to get your family to eat more fibre.

½ cup	peanut butter (natural, no sugar added)
⅓ cup	soft non-hydrogenated margarine
½ cup	brown sugar substitute
1	egg
2 tsp	vanilla
½ tsp	each baking soda and baking powder
Pinch	salt
1 cup	crushed All-Bran or Bran Buds cereal
¼ cup	whole wheat flour

1. In large bowl, using electric mixer, beat together peanut butter and margarine. Add sugar substitute, egg, vanilla, baking soda and powder, and salt and beat until sticky. Stir in cereal and flour until combined.
2. Scoop out 1 tbsp dough and, using damp hands, roll into ball. Place on parchment paper–lined baking sheet and repeat with remaining dough, leaving 2 inches between each cookie. Using floured fork, flatten cookies slightly with tines of fork.
3. Bake in 375° F oven for about 10 minutes or until light brown on bottom. Let cookies cool on rack for 2 minutes. Transfer to rack to cool completely.

Makes about 18 cookies.

APPLE RASPBERRY COFFEE CAKE   GREEN-LIGHT

A piece of this fruit-laden cake makes a delectable light dessert. It can be refrigerated for up to three days.

1 cup	whole wheat flour
¹/₂ cup	wheat bran
¹/₂ cup	brown sugar substitute
1 ¹/₂ tsp	baking powder
¹/₂ tsp	baking soda
¹/₄ tsp	cinnamon
¹/₄ tsp	ground nutmeg
Pinch	salt
¹/₂ cup	buttermilk
¹/₄ cup	soft non-hydrogenated margarine, melted and cooled
¹/₄ cup	liquid eggs
2 tsp	vanilla
1 cup	fresh raspberries
1	apple, cored and diced

Topping:

¹/₃ cup	large-flake rolled oats
¹/₄ cup	brown sugar substitute
2 tbsp	chopped pecans
1 tbsp	soft non-hydrogenated margarine

1. In large bowl, whisk together flour, bran, brown sugar substitute, baking powder and soda, cinnamon, nutmeg and salt; set aside.

2. In another bowl, whisk together buttermilk, margarine, liquid eggs and vanilla. Pour over flour mixture and stir until moistened. Spread two-thirds of the batter into parchment paper–lined 8-inch baking pan. Toss raspberries and apple together and sprinkle over batter. Dollop with remaining batter and spread gently with wet spatula.

3. **Topping:** In bowl, mix together oats, brown sugar substitute, pecans and margarine until combined. Sprinkle over top of cake; press gently into batter. Bake in 350° F oven for about 30 minutes or until tester inserted in centre comes out clean.

Makes 9 servings.

Appendix I

The Complete G.I. Diet Food Guide

BEANS		
Baked beans with pork		Baked beans* (low-fat)
Broad		Black beans
Refried		Black-eyed peas
		Butter beans
		Chickpeas
		Italian
		Lentils
		Mung
		Navy
		Pigeon
		Romano
		Soybeans
		Split peas

* Limit serving size (see page 27).

BEVERAGES

Alcoholic drinks*	Diet soft drinks (caffeinated)	Bottled water
Fruit drinks		Club soda
Milk (whole or 2%)	Milk (1%)	Decaffeinated coffee (with skim milk, no sugar)
Regular coffee	Most unsweetened juice	
Regular soft drinks		
Sweetened juice	Red wine*	Diet soft drinks (no caffeine)
Watermelon juice	Vegetable juices	
		Herbal tea
		Light instant chocolate
		Milk (skim)
		Soy milk (plain, low fat)
		Tea (with skim milk, no sugar)

BREADS

Bagels	Crispbreads (with fibre)*	100% stone-ground whole wheat*
Baguette/ Croissants	Pita (whole wheat)	Crispbreads (with high fibre, e.g., Wasa Fibre)*
Cake/Cookies	Tortillas (whole wheat)	
Cornbread		Green-light muffins (see pp. 274–77)
Crispbreads (regular)	Whole grain breads	
Croutons		Homemade Applesauce Bars (see p. 272–73)
English muffins		
Hamburger buns		Whole grain, high-fibre breads (2½– 3 g fibre per slice)*
Hot dog buns		
Kaiser rolls		
Melba toast		
Muffins/Doughnuts		

* Limit serving size (see page 27).

Pancakes/Waffles		
Pizza		
Stuffing		
Tortillas		
White bread		

CEREALS

All cold cereals except those listed as yellow- or green-light	Kashi Go Lean Crunch	100% Bran
		All-Bran
	Kashi Good Friends	Bran Buds
	Red River	Fibre 1
Cereal/Granola bars	Shredded Wheat Bran	Fibre First
Granola		Kashi Go Lean
Grits		Oat Bran
Muesli (commercial)		Porridge (old-fashioned rolled oats)

CEREAL/GRAINS

Amaranth	Cornstarch	Arrowroot flour
Couscous	Spelt	Barley
Millet		Buckwheat
Polenta		Bulgur
Rice (short-grain, white, instant)		Kamut (not puffed)
		Quinoa
Rice cakes		Rice (basmati, wild, brown, long-grain)
		Wheat berries

CONDIMENTS/SEASONINGS

Ketchup	Mayonnaise (light)	Capers
Mayonnaise		Extracts (vanilla, etc.)
Tartar sauce		Garlic

		Gravy mix (maximum 20 calories per 1/4 cup serving)
		Herbs and spices
		Horseradish
		Hummus
		Mayonnaise (fat-free)
		Mustard
		Salsa (no added sugar)
		Sauerkraut
		Soy sauce (low sodium)
		Teriyaki sauce
		Vinegar
		Worcestershire sauce

DAIRY

Almond milk	Cheese (low-fat)	Buttermilk
Cheese	Cream cheese (light)	Cheese (fat-free)
Chocolate milk		Cottage cheese (1% or fat-free)
Coconut milk	Frozen yogurt (low-fat, low sugar)	
Cottage cheese (whole or 2%)	Ice cream (low-fat)	Extra low-fat cheese (e.g., Laughing Cow Light, Boursin Light)
Cream	Milk (1%)	
Cream cheese	Sour cream (light)	
Evaporated milk	Yogurt (low-fat, with sugar)	Fruit yogurt (non-fat with sugar substitute)
Goat milk		
Ice cream		
Milk (whole or 2%)		

Rice milk		Ice cream (low-fat and no added sugar, e.g., Breyers Premium Fat Free, Nestlé Legend
Sour cream		
Yogurt (whole or 2%)		
		Milk (skim)
		Soy milk (plain, low-fat)
		Soy cheese (low-fat)

FATS AND OILS

Butter	Corn oil	Almonds*
Coconut oil	Mayonnaise (light)	Canola oil*/seed
Hard margarine	Most nuts	Cashews*
Lard	Natural nut butters	Flax seed
Mayonnaise	Natural peanut butter	Hazelnuts*
Palm oil	Peanuts	Macadamia nuts*
Peanut butter (regular and light)	Peanut oil	Mayonnaise (fat-free)
	Pecans	Olive oil*
Salad dressings (regular)	Salad dressings (light)	Pistachios*
Tropical oils	Sesame oil	Salad dressings (low-fat, low sugar)
Vegetable shortening	Soft margarine (non-hydrogenated)	Soft margarine (non-hydrogenated, light)*
	Sunflower oil	
	Vegetable oils	Vegetable oil sprays
	Walnuts	

* **Limit serving size (see page 27).**

FRUITS			
FRESH	Cantaloupe	Apricots	Apples
	Honeydew melon	Bananas	Avocado*
	Watermelon	Custard apples	Blackberries
		Figs	Blueberries
		Kiwi	Cherries
		Mango	Cranberries
		Papaya	Grapefruit
		Pineapple	Grapes
		Pomegranates	Guavas
			Lemons
			Oranges (all varieties)
			Peaches/Nectarines
			Plums
			Pears
			Raspberries
			Rhubarb
			Strawberries
BOTTLED, CANNED, DRIED, FROZEN	All canned fruit in syrup	Canned apricots in juice or water	Applesauce (without sugar)
	Applesauce containing sugar	Dried apples	Frozen berries
	Most dried fruit**	Dried apricots**	Fruit spreads (double fruit, no added sugar)
		Dried cranberries**	
		Fruit cocktail in juice	Mandarin oranges
		Peaches/Pears in syrup	Peaches/Pears in juice or water

*Limit serving size (see page 27).

** For baking, it is OK to use a modest amount of dried apricots or cranberries.

JUICES*		
Fruit drinks	Apple (unsweetened)	
Prune	Cranberry (unsweetened)	
Sweetened juice	Grapefruit (unsweetened)	
Watermelon	Orange (unsweetened)	
	Pear (unsweetened)	
	Pineapple (unsweetened)	
	Vegetable	

MEAT, POULTRY, FISH, EGGS AND TOFU		
Beef (brisket, short ribs)	Beef (sirloin steak, sirloin tip)	All fish and seafood, fresh, frozen or canned (in water)
Bologna	Chicken/Turkey leg (skinless)	Back bacon
Breaded fish and seafood	Corn beef	Beef (top/eye round steak)
Duck	Dried beef	Chicken breast (skinless)
Fish canned in oil	Flank steak	Egg whites
Goose	Ground beef (lean)	Ground beef (extra lean)
Ground beef (more than 10% fat)	Lamb (fore/leg shank, centre cut loin chop)	Lean deli ham
Hamburgers	Pork (centre loin, fresh ham, shank, sirloin, top loin)	Liquid eggs
Hot dogs		Pastrami (turkey)
Lamb (rack)	Turkey bacon	Pork tenderloin
Organ meats	Whole omega-3 eggs	Sashimi
Pastrami (beef)	Tofu	Soy cheese (low-fat)
Pâté		Tofu (low-fat)
Pork (back ribs, blade, spare ribs)		

* Whenever possible, eat the fruit rather than drink its juice.

Regular bacon		Turkey breast (skinless)
Salami		Turkey roll
Sausages		TVP (Textured Vegetable Protein)
Sushi		
Whole regular eggs		Veal
		Veggie burger
		Venison

PASTA

All canned pastas	Rice noodles	Capellini
Gnocchi		Fettuccine
Macaroni and cheese		Macaroni
Noodles (canned or instant)		Mung bean noodles
		Penne
Pasta filled with cheese or meat		Rigatoni
		Spaghetti/Linguine
		Vermicelli

PASTA SAUCES

Alfredo	Sauces with vegetables (no added sugar)	Light sauces with vegetables (no added sugar, e.g., Healthy Choice)
Sauces with added meat or cheese		
Sauces with added sugar or sucrose		

SNACKS

Bagels	Bananas	Almonds*
Candy	Dark chocolate* (70% cocoa)	Applesauce (unsweetened)
Cookies		
Crackers	Ice cream (low-fat)	Canned peaches/pears in juice or water
Doughnuts	Most nuts*	
Flavoured gelatin (all varieties)	Popcorn (air popped)	Cottage cheese (1% or fat-free)

* Limit serving size (see page 27).

French fries	Extra low-fat cheese (e.g., Laughing Cow Light, Boursin Light)
Ice cream	
Muffins (commercial)	Fruit yogurt (non-fat with sugar substitute)
Popcorn (regular)	
Potato chips	Food bars*
Pretzels	Green-light muffins (see pp. 274–77)
Pudding	
Raisins	Hazelnuts**
Rice cakes	Homemade Applesauce Bars (see p. 272–73)
Sorbet	
Tortilla chips	Ice cream (low-fat and no added sugar, e.g., Breyers Premium Fat Free, Nestlé Legend)
Trail mix	
White bread	
	Most fresh fruit
	Most fresh vegetables
	Most seeds
	Pickles
	Sugar-free hard candies

* **180–225 calorie bars, e.g., Zone or Balance Bars; 1/2 bar per serving**
** **Limit serving size (see page 27).**

SOUPS

All cream-based soups	Canned chicken noodle	Chunky bean and vegetable soups (e.g., Campbell's Healthy Request, Healthy Choice, and Too Good To Be True)
Canned black bean	Canned lentil	
Canned green pea	Canned tomato	
Canned puréed vegetable		
Canned split pea		Homemeade soups with green-light ingredients

SUGAR & SWEETENERS

Corn syrup	Fructose	Aspartame
Glucose	Sugar alcohols	Equal
Honey		Splenda
Molasses		Stevia (note: not FDA approved)
Sugar (all types)		Sugar Twin
		Sweet'N Low

VEGETABLES

Broad beans	Artichokes	Alfalfa sprouts	Cauliflower
French fries	Beets	Asparagus	Celery
Hash browns	Corn	Beans (green/wax)	Collard greens
Parsnips	Potatoes (boiled)	Bell peppers	Cucumbers
Potatoes (instant)	Pumpkin	Bok choy	Eggplant
Potatoes (mashed or baked)	Squash	Broccoli	Hearts of palm
	Sweet potatoes	Brussels sprouts	Kale
Rutabaga	Yams	Cabbage (all varieties)	Kohlrabi
Turnip		Carrots	Lettuce
			Mushrooms

		Mustard greens	Radicchio
		Okra	Radishes
		Olives*	Rapini
		Onions	Snow peas
		Peas	Spinach
		Peppers (hot)	Swiss chard
		Pickles	Tomatoes
		Potatoes (boiled, new)*	Zucchini

* Limit serving size (see page 27).

Appendix II

G.I. Diet Shopping List

PANTRY	FRIDGE/FREEZER
BAKING/COOKING	**DAIRY**
Baking powder/soda	Cottage cheese (1%)
Cocoa	Ice cream (low-fat, no added sugar)
Dried apricots	Milk (skim)
Sliced almonds	Sour cream (fat-free or 1%)
Wheat/oat bran	Soy milk (plain, low-fat)
Whole wheat flour	Yogurt (non-fat with sugar substitute)
BEANS (CANNED)	**FRUIT**
Baked beans (low-fat)	Apples
Mixed salad beans	Blueberries
BREAD	Cherries
100% stone-ground whole wheat	Grapefruit
CEREALS	Grapes
All-Bran	Lemons
Bran Buds	Limes
Fibre First	Oranges
Kashi Go Lean	Peaches
Oatmeal (old-fashioned rolled oats)	Pears

DRINKS	Plums
Bottled water	Strawberries
Decaffeinated coffee	**MEAT/POULTRY/FISH/EGGS**
Diet soft drinks	All fish and seafood (no breading)
Tea	Chicken/Turkey breast (skinless)
FATS/OILS	Extra-lean ground beef
Almonds	Lean deli style ham/turkey/chicken
Canola oil	Liquid eggs (Break Free/Omega Pro)
Margarine (non-hydrogenated, light)	Pork tenderloin
Mayonnaise (fat-free)	Veal
Olive oil	**VEGETABLES**
Salad dressings (fat-free)	Asparagus
Vegetable oil spray	Beans (green/wax)
FRUIT (CANNED/BOTTLED)	Bell and hot peppers
Applesauce (no sugar)	Broccoli
Mandarin oranges	Cabbage
Peaches in juice or water	Carrots
Pears in juice or water	Cauliflower
PASTA	Celery
Fettuccine	Cucumber
Macaroni	Eggplant
Penne	Lettuce
Spaghetti	Mushrooms
PASTA SAUCES	Olives
(vegetable-based only)	Onions
Healthy Choice	Pickles
Too Good To Be True	Potatoes (small, new only)
RICE	Spinach
Basmati/long-grain/wild	Tomatoes
SEASONINGS	Zucchini
Flavoured vinegars/sauces	**SOUPS**
Spices/herbs	Healthy Choice
Food bars (Zone/Balance)	Too Good To Be True
	SWEETENERS
	Equal, Splenda, Sweet'N Low, Sugar Twin (and other sugar substitutes)

Appendix III

Exercise Calorie Counter

WEIGHT (IN LB):	130	160	200
TIME (IN MIN):	30	30	30
GYM AND HOME ACTIVITIES			
Aerobics: low impact	172	211	264
Aerobics: high impact	218	269	336
Aerobics, Step: low impact	218	269	336
Aerobics, Step: high impact	312	384	480
Aerobics: water	125	154	192
Bicycling, Stationary: moderate	218	269	336
Bicycling, Stationary: vigorous	328	403	504
Circuit Training: general	250	307	384
Rowing, Stationary: moderate	218	269	336
Rowing, Stationary: vigorous	265	326	408
Ski Machine: general	296	365	456
Stair Step Machine: general	187	230	288
Weightlifting: general	94	115	144
Weightlifting: vigorous	187	230	288

TRAINING ACTIVITIES			
Basketball: playing a game	250	307	384
Basketball: wheelchair	203	250	312
Bicycling: BMX or mountain	265	326	408
Bicycling: 12–13.9 mph	250	307	384
Bicycling: 14–15.9 mph	312	384	480
Boxing: sparring	281	346	432
Football: competitive	281	346	432
Football: touch, flag, general	250	307	384
Frisbee	94	115	144
Golf: carrying clubs	172	211	264
Golf: using cart	109	134	168
Gymnastics: general	125	154	192
Handball: general	374	461	576
Hiking: cross-country	187	230	288
Horseback Riding: general	125	154	192
Ice Skating: general	218	269	336
Martial Arts: general	312	384	480
Racquetball: competitive	312	384	480
Racquetball: casual, general	218	269	336
Rock Climbing: ascending	343	422	528
Rock Climbing: repelling	250	307	384
Rollerblading	218	269	336
Rope Jumping	312	384	480
Running: 5 mph (12 min/mile)	250	307	384
Running: 5.2 mph (11.5 min/mile)	281	346	432
Running: 6 mph (10 min/mile)	312	384	480
Running: 6.7 mph (9 min/mile)	343	422	528
Running: 7.5 mph (8 min/mile)	390	480	600
Running: 8.6 mph (7 min/mile)	452	557	696
Running: 10 mph (6 min/mile)	515	634	792

Running: pushing wheelchair, marathon wheeling	250	307	384
Running: cross-country	281	346	432
Skiing: cross-country	250	307	384
Skiing: downhill	187	230	288
Snowshoeing	250	307	384
Softball: general play	156	192	240
Swimming: general	187	230	288
Tennis: general	218	269	336
Volleyball: non-competitive, general play	94	115	144
Volleyball: competitive, gymnasium play	125	154	192
Volleyball: beach	250	307	384
Walk: 3.5 mph (17 min/mile)	125	154	192
Walk: 4 mph (15 min/mile)	140	173	216
Walk: 4.5 mph (13 min/mile)	156	192	240
Walk/Jog: jog more than 10 min.	187	230	288
Water Polo	312	384	480
Waterskiing	187	230	288
Whitewater: rafting, kayaking	156	192	240
DAILY LIFE ACTIVITIES			
Children's Games: 4-square, etc.	156	192	240
Chopping & Splitting Wood	187	230	288
Gardening: general	140	173	216
Housecleaning: general	109	134	168
Mowing Lawn: push, hand	172	211	264
Mowing Lawn: push, power	140	173	216
Operate Snow Blower: walking	140	173	216
Raking Lawn	125	154	192
Sex: moderate effort	47	58	72
Shovelling Snow: by hand	187	230	288

Appendix IV

Children's BMI Tables

Determining a child's BMI is a bit more complex than looking up an adult's, because children are still growing and obviously don't have a fixed height. The first step is to look up your child's height in the left vertical column of the Children's BMI Calculator on pages 302-03. Move across the chart until you reach your child's weight. The number at the top of that column is your child's BMI.

The next step is to determine how your child's BMI compares with others in the same age range. Because boys and girls mature at different rates, they require separate charts. For boys, use the chart on page 304; for girls, use the chart on page 305. Find your child's age along the bottom of the chart, and move up that line until you reach your child's BMI, which is indicated in the left vertical column. The point where those two lines intersect is the percentile into which your child fits, which is indicated on the right hand side of the chart. A percentile above 95 indicates overweight. A percentile between 85 and 95 indicates risk of becoming overweight. And a percentile under 5 indicates underweight. Let's look at an example: Jake is ten years old. He weighs 87 pounds and is 4 feet 6 inches. The Children's BMI Calculator tells us Jake has a BMI of 21. Now we look at the Boys' Body Mass Index-for-Age Percentiles chart on page 304. We find Jake's age, ten years along the bottom of the chart, and move up that line until we come to a BMI of 21. Jake is somewhere between the 90th and 95th percentile, which indicates he is at risk of becoming overweight.

Let's look at another example: Emily is seven years old, weighs 52 pounds and is 4 feet tall. Based on the Children's BMI Calculator, her BMI is 16. Checking the Girls' Body Mass Index-for-Age Percentiles chart on page 305, we see that her percentile falls between 50 and 75, which puts her well within the normal range.

Note: These guidelines are only one way of determining if your child is at risk. Always check with your pediatrician or doctor before making any major dietary decisions regarding your child.

CHILDREN'

Ht (in.)	BMI 13	14	15	16	17	18	19	20	21	22
32	19	20	22	23	25	26	28	29	31	32
33	20	22	23	25	26	28	29	31	33	34
34	21	23	25	26	28	30	31	33	35	36
35	23	24	26	28	30	31	33	35	37	38
36	24	26	28	29	31	33	35	37	39	41
37	25	27	29	31	33	35	37	39	41	43
38	27	29	31	33	35	37	39	41	43	45
39	28	30	32	35	37	39	41	43	45	48
40	30	32	34	36	39	41	43	46	48	50
41	31	33	36	38	41	43	45	48	50	53
42	33	35	38	40	43	45	48	50	53	55
43	34	37	39	42	45	47	50	53	55	58
44	36	39	41	44	47	50	52	55	58	61
45	37	40	43	46	49	52	55	58	60	63
46	39	42	45	48	51	54	57	60	63	66
47	41	44	47	50	53	57	60	63	66	69
48	43	46	49	52	56	59	62	66	69	72
49	44	48	51	55	58	61	65	68	72	75
50	46	50	53	57	60	64	68	71	75	78
51	48	52	55	59	63	67	70	74	78	81
52	50	54	58	62	65	69	73	77	81	85
53	52	56	60	64	68	72	76	80	84	88
54	54	58	62	66	71	75	79	83	87	91
55	56	60	65	69	73	77	82	86	90	95
56	58	62	67	71	76	80	85	89	94	98
57	60	65	69	74	79	83	88	92	97	102
58	62	67	72	77	81	86	91	96	100	105
59	64	69	74	79	84	89	94	99	104	109
60	67	72	77	82	87	92	97	102	108	113
61	69	74	79	85	90	95	101	106	111	116
62	71	77	82	87	93	98	104	109	115	120
63	73	79	85	90	96	102	107	113	119	124
64	76	82	87	93	99	105	111	117	122	128
65	78	84	90	96	102	108	114	120	126	132
66	81	87	93	99	105	112	118	124	130	136
67	83	89	96	102	109	115	121	128	134	140
68	86	92	99	105	112	118	125	132	138	145
69	88	95	102	108	115	122	129	135	142	149
70	91	98	105	112	118	125	132	139	146	153
71	93	100	108	115	122	129	136	143	151	158
72	96	103	111	118	125	133	140	147	155	162

MI CALCULATOR

24	25	26	27	28	29	30	31	32	33	34	35
35	36	38	39	41	42	44	45	47	48	50	51
37	39	40	42	43	45	46	48	50	51	53	54
39	41	43	44	46	48	49	51	53	54	56	58
42	44	45	47	49	51	52	54	56	58	59	61
44	46	48	50	52	53	55	57	59	61	63	65
47	49	51	53	55	56	58	60	62	64	66	68
49	51	53	55	58	60	62	64	66	68	70	72
52	54	56	58	61	63	65	67	69	71	74	76
55	57	59	61	64	66	68	71	73	75	77	80
57	60	62	65	67	69	72	74	77	79	81	84
60	63	65	68	70	73	75	78	80	83	85	88
63	66	68	71	74	76	79	82	84	87	89	92
66	69	72	74	77	80	83	85	88	91	94	96
69	72	75	78	81	84	86	89	92	95	98	101
72	75	78	81	84	87	90	93	96	99	102	105
75	79	82	85	88	91	94	97	101	104	107	110
79	82	85	88	92	95	98	102	105	108	111	115
82	85	89	92	96	99	102	106	109	113	116	120
85	89	92	96	100	103	107	110	114	117	121	124
89	92	96	100	104	107	111	115	118	122	126	129
92	96	100	104	108	112	115	119	123	127	131	135
96	100	104	108	112	116	120	124	128	132	136	140
100	104	108	112	116	120	124	129	133	137	141	145
103	108	112	116	120	125	129	133	138	142	146	151
107	112	116	120	125	129	134	138	143	147	152	156
111	116	120	125	129	134	139	143	148	153	157	162
115	120	124	129	134	139	144	148	153	158	163	167
119	124	129	134	139	144	149	154	158	163	168	173
123	128	133	138	143	149	154	159	164	169	174	179
127	132	138	143	148	153	159	164	169	175	180	185
131	137	142	148	153	159	164	170	175	180	186	191
135	141	147	152	158	164	169	175	181	186	192	198
140	146	151	157	163	169	175	181	186	192	198	204
144	150	156	162	168	174	180	186	192	198	204	210
149	155	161	167	173	180	186	192	198	204	211	217
153	160	166	172	179	185	192	198	204	211	217	223
158	164	171	178	184	191	197	204	210	217	224	230
163	169	176	183	190	196	203	210	217	223	230	237
167	174	181	188	195	202	209	216	223	230	237	244
172	179	186	194	201	208	215	222	229	237	244	251
177	184	192	199	206	214	221	229	236	243	251	258

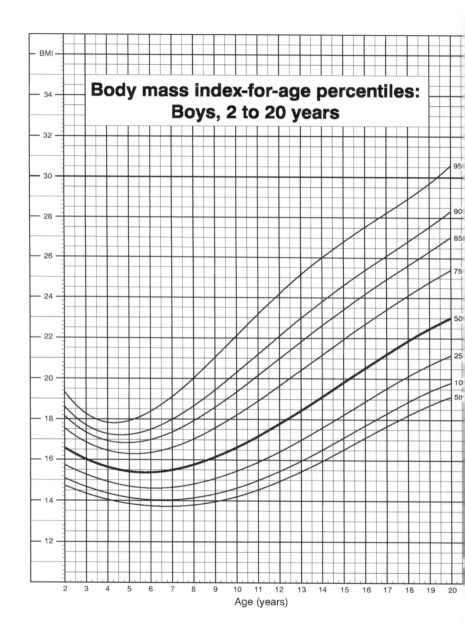

Body mass index-for-age percentiles: Boys, 2 to 20 years

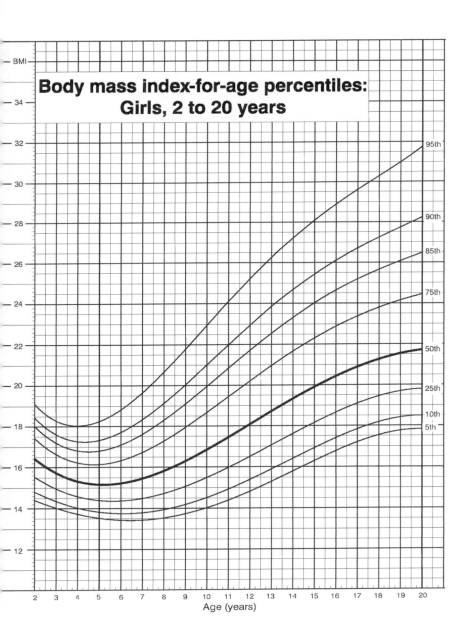

BMI

34

32 — 95th

30

28 — 90th

— 85th

26

— 75th

24

22 — 50th

20 — 25th

— 10th
18 — 5th

16

14

12

Body mass index-for-age percentiles:
Girls, 2 to 20 years

2   3   4   5   6   7   8   9   10 11 12 13 14 15 16 17 18 19 20
Age (years)

Appendix V

The Ten Golden G.I. Diet Rules

1. Eat three meals and three snacks every day. Don't skip meals—particularly breakfast.

2. Stick with green-light products only in Phase I.

3. When it comes to food, quantity is as important as quality. Shrink your usual portions, particularly of meat, pasta and rice.

4. Always ensure that each meal contains the appropriate measure of carbohydrates, protein and fat.

5. Eat at least three times more vegetables and fruit than usual.

6. Drink plenty of fluids, preferably water.

7. Exercise for thirty minutes once a day or fifteen minutes twice a day. Get off the bus three stops early.

8. Find a friend to join you for mutual support.

9. Set realistic goals. Try to lose an average of a pound a week and record your progress to reinforce your sense of achievement.

10. Don't view this as a diet. It's the basis of how you will eat for the rest of your life.

G.I. DIET WEEKLY WEIGHT/WAIST LOG

WEEK	DATE	WEIGHT	WAIST	COMMENTS
1.				
2.				
3.				
4.				
5.				
6.				
7.				
8.				
9.				
10.				
11.				
12.				
13.				
14.				
15.				
16.				
17.				
18.				
19.				
20.				

Acknowledgements

My thanks to the readers of *The G.I. Diet* as they have been the inspiration for this book. I have received literally thousands of emails expressing interest or concern over managing the whole family's nutrition and health. As most of the writers were women, we have endeavoured to address these issues through their eyes. Nutrition and health truly are a family affair.

On a more personal note, my editor Stacey Cameron has been a constant cheerleader and a tremendous support through the lengthy process of bringing this book into print.

Index

Page references in italics indicate recipes

Recipe Index